All About
ANAESTHESIA

Jan Davies and Rod Westhorpe

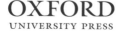
OXFORD
UNIVERSITY PRESS

OXFORD
UNIVERSITY PRESS

253 Normanby Road, South Melbourne, Victoria, Australia

Oxford University Press is a department of the University of Oxford.
It furthers the University's objective of excellence in research, scholarship,
and education by publishing worldwide in

Oxford New York

Athens Auckland Bangkok Bogotá
Buenos Aires Calcutta Cape Town Chennai
Dar es Salaam Delhi Florence Hong Kong
Istanbul Karachi Kuala Lumpur Madrid Melbourne
Mexico City Mumbai Nairobi Paris Port Moresby
São Paulo Shanghai Singapore Taipei Tokyo Toronto Warsaw

and associated companies in
Berlin Ibadan

OXFORD is a trade mark of Oxford University Press

National Library of Australia
Cataloguing-in-publication data:

Davies, Jan.
All about anaesthesia.

Bibliography.
Includes index.
ISBN 0 19 551089 5.

1. Anaesthesia. I. Westhorpe, Rod. II. Title.

617.96

Edited by Janet Mackenzie
Illustrated by Vasja Koman
Indexed by Russell Brooks
Text and cover designed by Karen Trump
Cover photograph from PhotoDisk
Typeset by Solo Typesetting, Adelaide
Printed through Bookpac Production Services, Singapore

Contents

Figures

Introduction

Most people experience an anaesthetic at some time in their lives, and some undergo anaesthesia many times. It is normal for people to be uneasy about having an anaesthetic; however, modern anaesthesia is very safe and, indeed, modern surgery would not be possible without developments in anaesthesia.

The aim of this book is to explain what anaesthesia is, describe how anaesthetics are given, and detail how anaesthetists care for you. We also show how anaesthetics can affect you and how you can affect your anaesthetic. Much of this information comes from following the course of seven patients as they make their way to and from the Operating Room. The questions they ask and the answers they receive supplement basic descriptions of every part of the process of undergoing anaesthesia for surgery or other procedures.

In chapter 1 we introduce you to the specialty of anaesthesia. We describe who gives anaesthetics, their training, and the different terms applied to anaesthetists in English-speaking countries. We also outline the types of work they carry out, and detail how and why anaesthesia today is safe. In the second chapter, we explain how an anaesthetic is not 'just a needle'. In chapter 3 we introduce you to your fellow patients. Chapter 4 discusses the different options for different patients, including an explanation of informed consent. In chapter 5 we detail how you are evaluated before an anaesthetic. This evaluation includes your general health and also aspects of your condition specific to the reason for undergoing anaesthesia. How you are prepared for an anaesthetic is the subject of chapter 6. Again, both general preparation and preparation specific to anaesthesia are included. The next two chapters describe what happens as you undergo an anaesthetic (chapter 7) and afterwards (chapter 8). In chapters 9 and 10 we recount common patient fears and complaints. Chapter 11 describes possible complications of anaesthesia. The last chapter gives suggestions as to what you should do if you think that something has gone wrong.

Appendix 1 provides details of what you can do to help, such as not smoking, and following the instructions given by your anaesthetist, your surgeon, and other professionals looking after you. In Appendix 2 we provide questions to ask your anaesthetist. There is also a Glossary, explaining each of the words from the text shown in italic type. The list of Further Information provides sources of information from the Internet that we think give sensible and sound advice to help you in making choices about the care you receive.

A note on pronunciation

In all of these words, the 'th' is pronounced as in 'think', not as in 'these':

- *anaesthesia* is pronounced 'an-ess-THEEZ-ya'
- *anaesthetic* is pronounced 'an-ess-THETT-ik'
- *anaesthetist* is pronounced 'an-ESS-the-tist' or 'an-EES-the-tist'
- *anaesthesiologist* and *anesthesiologist* are both pronounced 'AN-ess-THEEZ-ee-OL-o-jist'.

Chapter 1

Anaesthesia: what is it and is it safe?

Anaesthesia is a word derived from the Greek, meaning 'without sensation'. Anaesthesia may be applied to the whole body, when it is known as *general anaesthesia*, or to part of the body, when it is known as *regional* or *local anaesthesia*. All of these techniques involve giving specific drugs that interfere with the transmission of nervous impulses so as to reduce sensation. An *anaesthetic* is the term applied to some or all of the drugs used to produce anaesthesia and is also used to describe the whole process. (For example, one might say, 'Mary had a general anaesthetic.')

We describe the people involved in anaesthesia and discuss the safety aspects.

WHO GIVES YOUR ANAESTHETIC?

If you live in Australia, Canada, New Zealand, South Africa, or the United Kingdom, your anaesthetic will most likely be given by a specialist doctor. Depending on the country, this specialist is known as the *anaesthetist* or *anaesthesiologist* or *anesthesiologist*.

After graduating from medical school, these doctors have undertaken several years' additional training in anaesthesia. Anaesthetic training is usually under the direction of a professional body, such as the Australian and New Zealand College of Anaesthetists, the Royal College of Physicians and Surgeons of Canada, or the Royal College of Anaesthetists in the United Kingdom. The training varies in content and length, depending on the country in which it is undertaken. In those countries mentioned above, the training is for a minimum of several years and equal in length to that of other specialists, including surgeons. The process to become a specialist anaesthetist includes intensive assessment and written and oral examinations. If successful in passing the examinations, the anaesthetist becomes a Fellow of the national professional accrediting body, such as one of the colleges mentioned above.

In Canada and the United States of America, specialist anaesthetists are known as anesthesiologists. American anesthesiologists have always been known by this term, to distinguish these doctors from Certified Registered Nurse Anesthetists or CRNAs (see below). In 1998, Canadian anaesthetists decided to change their designation also to anesthesiologists, because of the confusion with American nurse anesthetists. There are no nurse anaesthetists practising in Canada, Australia, New Zealand, or the United Kingdom.

In the United States, at the completion of anaesthetic training, the doctor takes a written examination. The successful candidate must then pass an oral examination to become a Board Certified anesthesiologist. In Europe and many other countries, specialist anaesthetists are known as anaesthesiologists. This again denotes the distinction from 'nurse anaesthetists' who practise with specialists in many European countries.

After qualification, anaesthetists are strongly encouraged to continue their education throughout their professional lives. Most colleges or other regulatory and licensing bodies now require some ongoing evidence that the anaesthetist is keeping up to date. The degree of professional regulation depends on the country in which the anaesthetist practises.

In Canada, the Canadian Anesthesiologists' Society is a professional organisation that has undertaken development of *Guidelines to the Practice of Anaesthesia*. These provide recommendations as to how anaesthetics are given—for example, which *monitors* should be used during an anaesthetic. The Royal College of Physicians and Surgeons of Canada (RCPSC), which regulates training and certification of anesthesiologists, plays no further specific role in the regulation of anaesthetic practice. However, the RCPSC does direct a system of continuing medical education, known as Maintenance of Competence.

By way of contrast, in Australia and New Zealand, the College of Anaesthetists (ANZCA) has developed guidelines for anaesthetic practice. In addition, the college directs a Maintenance of Professional Standards program in which any anaesthetist can participate.

In some countries, non-specialist doctors may also give anaes-thetics, most often in rural areas. Smaller communities depend on non-specialist anaesthetists because the amount of work available is not sufficient to support a full-time specialist. Although only one specialist might be needed for the normal or *elective* work, that specialist would also have to be on call for emergencies all the time—seven days a week and 52 weeks a year. Obviously this is not an ideal situation and so the needs of a community are usually met by non-specialists. These doctors have not had full specialty training. Depending on where they practise, the require-ments for training vary greatly in content and length. In general, non-specialist anaesthetists tend to give anaesthetics for less com-plex operations. Many non-specialists anaesthetists also continue to work as family or general practitioners.

Non-medical practitioners

In some countries, particularly in Europe, nurse anaesthetists give anaesthetics under the supervision of a specialist anaesthesiologist. Often they work as a team, with one nurse anaesthetist and one anaesthesiologist for each patient. In other areas, nurse anaesthetists give anaesthetics under the direction of the surgeon, *cardiologist*, or *radiologist* who is operating or performing a procedure on a patient at the same time. In a few countries, nurse anaesthetists are legally allowed to practise without any supervision by a doctor.

Other assistants

In the Operating Room, your anaesthetist usually has the help of an assistant. This person could be a nurse, a *respiratory therapist*, or an *anaesthetic technician*. Ideally, the assistant has undergone formal training and examination, although this is not always the case. Anaesthetists value good assistants, who carry out many differing tasks. These tasks include preparing and checking drugs and equipment, and obtaining extra equipment from outside the Operating Room. The assistant may also attach various monitors to you, such as an automatic blood pressure cuff, and then may record your heart rate, blood pressure, and other measurements on the *anaesthetic record*. In addition, the assistant hands drugs or equipment to your anaesthetist, and is generally available to help at all times, particularly at the beginning and end of the anaesthetic.

Depending on where you live and where your hospital is, a number of the people described above may be involved in providing your anaesthetic care. In addition, some hospitals also train other health care workers, such as ambulance attendants and paramedics, who may be present in the Operating Room and help with part of your anaesthetic.

WHAT TYPES OF WORK DO ANAESTHETISTS DO?

Anaesthetists provide anaesthetic care for surgical operations, before the operation (*preoperative*), during the operation (*intraoperative*), and after the operation (*postoperative*). They also provide anaesthetic care for patients undergoing non-surgical procedures, such as special heart examinations or X-ray treatment, particularly if these procedures are long, complex, or painful. Sometimes this care consists of providing *sedation*, either for a procedure such as an examination of the bowel (*endoscopy*) or in addition to regional or local anaesthesia. (This is often called *monitored anaesthesia care*.)

In addition, anaesthetists provide relief of *acute pain* for women during labour and delivery, and to many patients after operations, as well as treatment of *chronic pain* for patients with long-term pain problems. Many anaesthetists are involved in intensive care or in the provision of retrieval services and resuscitation. Retrieval services involve going by air or road ambulance to fetch accident victims or patients from a small hospital who need specialised care in a major hospital. Other anaesthetists spend part of their time doing research in diverse fields – studying how the body works, developing new drugs and equipment, and working out how to teach teams of medical workers to minimise human error and accidents.

Many anaesthetists also teach a wide range of health care workers, including medical and nursing students, interns, residents, specialists in training, and other specialists (surgeons, *obstetricians*, *physicians*, etc.). Anaesthetists are often asked to give talks of a general nature to interested groups, such as the Scouts, community organisations, and school classes. (If you would like to have an anaesthetist speak to your group, contact your local hospital Department of Anaesthesia or the College or Society.)

No matter which type of anaesthetic care they provide, the responsibilities of anaesthetists are similar. These responsibilities include evaluating the patient before the operation or procedure; forming a plan for the care of the patient during and after the anaesthetic; monitoring and supporting the patient during the procedure; and supervising care after the procedure.

IS ANAESTHESIA SAFE?

Modern anaesthesia is safe, despite some of the stories you hear. To compare one hour of being anaesthetised with, say, one hour spent in traffic or a one-hour plane trip, the risk of dying is about one in two million in traffic, about one in one million in an aircraft, and one in 100,000–500,000 during the anaesthetic. If you compare one hour of having an anaesthetic with an hour of air travel, then the risk of dying is about five to ten times higher during the anaesthetic. In contrast, an hour spent parachute-jumping carries a risk of death about 20–100 times that associated with anaesthesia.

The safety of anaesthesia has increased over the years, even though much more complicated operations are being performed. For example, in Australia, the risk of death associated with anaesthesia has decreased to one-tenth of what it was thirty years ago. You can be confident that modern anaesthesia is very safe.

What makes anaesthesia safe?

A number of factors have contributed to the overall safety of modern anaesthesia. These factors include your anaesthetist, the drugs and equipment used in the Operating Room, and overall medical care. For example, your anaesthetist is responsible for your overall health and safety from the start of your anaesthetic until you leave the *Recovery Room* after your operation. Your anaesthetist makes sure that all the anaesthetic equipment is working properly before you undergo anaesthesia. (This is just like the airline pilot who completes a pre-flight check of the aeroplane.) Your anaesthetist knows what to do if a problem occurs with any of the equipment during your anaesthetic. He or she will be with you throughout your operation, watching you and watching your surgeon. Your anaesthetist also continuously watches a number of monitors that measure many of the things happening to you while you are under the effects of the anaesthetic. Should there be any complications, either because of the anaesthetic drugs, or more likely because of the operation, your anaesthetist will respond quickly, having been fully trained in managing emergencies.

There have been major improvements in the drugs used for anaesthesia. Starting in 1846, the first anaesthetics were given with one drug, such as ether or chloroform. Inhaling these drugs was unpleasant, because of the smell and a sensation of choking. *Induction* of anaesthesia was often slow, and occasionally patients would struggle and have to be restrained. Because only one drug was used, patients needed heavy doses to make them very deeply anaesthetised. This was to ensure that the patients' muscles were sufficiently relaxed for the surgeons to be able to operate. After the operation, patients often slept for long periods of time, as they breathed out the large amounts of drug that had been used. Vomiting and severe postoperative pain were very common.

Since the 1940s, anaesthetists have had the benefit of being able to use many new anaesthetic agents. All have contributed to the development of anaesthetic practice as it is today. The newer agents tend to be absorbed less by the body's fat, which means that they have a shorter duration of action than the older agents. This allows anaesthetists to determine and control the depth of an anaesthetic more precisely for the requirements of each individual patient. However, the principle upon which the use of all of these drugs is based remains common to those of the original agents—'sufficient and safe'.

In addition to improvements in anaesthetic agents, there have been major changes in the equipment used to give the anaesthetic and to monitor its effects. As recently as the mid-1970s, anaesthetics were given in modern hospitals in Canada and Australia with only a blood pressure cuff and a stethoscope to monitor the patient. Since then, many new pieces of equipment have been introduced. As a result, anaesthetists are now better able to assess and evaluate what is happening to their patients.

A final word should be said about the cost of anaesthetic care, which is in addition to the cost of surgical care. Fees charged by anaesthetists for their services vary in different countries, and depend on whether or not medical treatment is covered by a public health system. For patients receiving private medical care, the fee varies according to the length and complexity of the anaesthetic. In Australia, fees range from around $100 to $2000 or more. If you live in a country where anaesthetic fees are charged, you should ask your anaesthetist about the fees before the procedure.

Chapter 2

Not just a needle

Many people think that having an anaesthetic consists of just a needle, which the anaesthetist injects to make you 'go to sleep'; after this the anaesthetist leaves you and you 'wake up' when the operation is over. In fact, while constantly looking after you during your anaesthetic, your anaesthetist gives you quite a few drugs— usually somewhere between three and fifteen—all for different reasons.

ANAESTHETIC DRUGS

There are four main types of drugs used in general anaesthesia:
- **induction agents** to produce unconsciousness
- **analgesics** to provide pain relief
- **muscle relaxants** to induce muscle relaxation
- **inhalational agents** to keep you unconscious.

Other drugs include those given to produce short-term memory loss or amnesia; to prevent nausea and vomiting (*anti-emetics*); to counteract the effect of other drugs (*antagonists*); and to suppress certain nervous reflexes, such as slowing of the heart. Some patients may not have a general anaesthetic but may remain conscious, with part of their body made numb by use of *local anaesthetics*.

Induction agents

These drugs include *thiopentone* or *Pentothal* (which was introduced in the 1930s), *propofol*, and ketamine. When given by intravenous injection, they act quickly to take you from being conscious to unconscious. This rapid loss of consciousness makes the induction of anaesthesia much more pleasant than previously, when patients had to breathe ether or chloroform.

Analgesics

These drugs, also known as painkillers, are mostly *narcotics*. They are either derived from the opium poppy (such as *morphine*) or synthesised in a laboratory (such as *pethidine* or *meperidine*, anileridine, fentanyl, alfentanil, sufentanil, and remifentanil).

Muscle relaxants

These drugs work specifically to weaken or relax most of the muscles of the body. However, they do not affect the muscles of the heart, nor those of the intestines. Before muscle relaxants were introduced in the 1940s, patients had to be given large amounts of anaesthetic drugs to ensure that they were deeply anaesthetised. This was necessary to cause their muscles to relax so that the surgeon could gain access to the abdomen. Now, with the use of muscle relaxants, patients do not have to receive very large amounts of anaesthetic drugs nor be so deeply anaesthetised. This helps to reduce the side-effects of anaesthesia. Muscle relaxants include suxamethonium (or succinyl choline), pancuronium, atracurium, vecuronium, and rocuronium.

Inhalational agents

These drugs keep you unconscious during the operation. They can also be used to induce anaesthesia, especially in small children. They are called inhalational agents because you inhale them or breathe them in. In the 1950s, a new inhalational agent, halothane, was introduced and rapidly replaced the older agents such as ether. Commonly used agents include enflurane, isoflurane, sevoflurane, and desflurane.

Anti-emetics

These drugs prevent or reduce nausea and vomiting. They are termed anti-nauseants or anti-emetics and include *droperidol*, Stemetil, Gravol, and ondansetron.

Other drugs

Your anaesthetist may use other drugs to decrease the chance of your remembering anything that happens in the Operating Room. These drugs include diazepam and midazolam, which belong to the class of drugs known as benzodiazepines.

Some drugs are given to counteract the effects of other drugs. These include naloxone, to counter the effects of a narcotic; flumazenil, to counter the effects of a benzodiazepine; and neo-stigmine, to reverse the actions of most of the muscle relaxants. Drugs which are used to change your heart rate include atropine (to increase it) and esmolol (to decrease it). Other drugs can raise your blood pressure (epinephrine or *adrenaline*) or lower it (nitro-prusside).

LOCAL ANAESTHETICS

Injection of a local anaesthetic around a nerve or a group of nerves blocks the transmission of the electrical impulses in the nerve. This causes the area of the body supplied by the nerve to become numb. This is also known as a 'sensory block', which may progress to muscle weakness, depending on the concentration and dose of the local anaesthetic used.

ANAESTHETIC EQUIPMENT

Some of the drugs given by the anaesthetist are injected, but others are inhaled. To deliver these inhaled drugs, as well as oxygen, your anaesthetist uses an *anaesthetic machine*.

What is the anaesthetic machine like?

The anaesthetic machine is not a machine that makes anaes-thetics, but a complex collection of equipment. It has three major components: a gas mixing and delivery system; an anaesthetic *breathing system* (circuit) and a *ventilator*; and an array of monitors. Some recently developed machines have highly complex integrated electronic systems and are usually called anaesthesia workstations.

The gas mixing and delivery system

The anaesthetic machine is connected to a supply of gases. These usually come from a bulk supply in the hospital or clinic, but sometimes from smaller compressed gas cylinders attached to the machine. All anaesthetic machines have cylinders to supply oxygen and nitrous oxide, and many also have a supply of compressed air. All the gases are purified and are supplied to the machine at a set pressure, usually around four times atmospheric pressure.

All the gases are mixed in a special device, which ensures accurate concentrations and limits the minimum amount of oxygen which can be used. To this gas mixture, the anaesthetist can add one of a range of additional, more powerful anaesthetic agents, known as inhalational agents. These come as a liquid and are placed in a device called a vaporiser, which converts them into a gas and adds them in carefully controlled concentrations to the gas mixture.

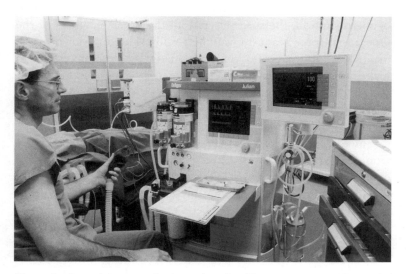

Figure 1   A modern anaesthetic workstation. There are two monitoring screens, one for gas and ventilation monitoring, and one for cardio-vascular and other patient data. There are two vaporisers, each specially calibrated for a particular inhalational anaesthetic agent.

The anaesthetic breathing system (circuit) and ventilator

The anaesthetist determines the flow rate of the final mixture of gases supplied to the breathing system. This is a series of hoses about three centimetres in diameter, which connect to either the mask or the *endotracheal tube*, and also to a ventilator. The breathing circuit is often attached to a container of 'soda lime' granules: these absorb carbon dioxide that the patient exhales with each breath.

The ventilator is an automatic breathing device, which takes over the rhythmic inflating and deflating of the patient's lungs in a programmed manner. The anaesthetist sets the gas flow, the oxygen concentration, the anaesthetic agent concentration, the amount of gas in each breath, and the number of breaths per minute.

The monitors

Some people think that anaesthetists do not do anything during an operation, once the anaesthetic has started. In fact, anaesthetists are very busy, watching and evaluating their patients, the progress of the operation, the surgeon, and all the other members of the Operating Room team. By watching and evaluating—or processing all this information—your anaesthetist is able, if necessary, to make moment-by-moment adjustments to the drugs and fluids that you need during your anaesthetic and operation. Your anaesthetist is also able to consider the plan for the next phases of your care, such as in the Recovery Room.

Some of the information that your anaesthetist evaluates comes from special monitors. Two kinds of monitors are used to make continuous checks. One set tells your anaesthetist all about you, including your heart rate, blood pressure, and temperature. The other set shows how the anaesthetic machine is functioning.

Measurements of how your body is reacting to the anaesthetic and operation or examination include:

- **Your heart rate (pulse) and rhythm:** by feeling the pulse in your wrist or your neck, by using a stethoscope to listen to your heart, and by means of an *electrocardiograph* (ECG or EKG). The same monitor can also be used to detect if your heart is suffering any strain.

- **Your (arterial) blood pressure:** by attaching a traditional inflatable cuff or sometimes by inserting a small tube or *cannula* (or catheter) directly into an artery.
- **The amount of oxygen in a small or peripheral artery:** by attaching a device like a clothes-peg, known as a *pulse oximeter*, to one of your fingers or toes or earlobes, or to the tip of your nose. The result is known as your *peripheral* arterial oxygen saturation.
- **The amount of carbon dioxide (CO_2) you breathe out:** by using a carbon dioxide detector. The result is known as your end-tidal (end of each breath) carbon dioxide concentration. This measurement helps your anaesthetist to check on the function of your lungs and on your metabolism. This monitor is also used to ensure that the breathing tube is correctly placed in your windpipe or *trachea* and that the breathing circuit has not become disconnected. (See below.)
- **How well you are breathing (or being breathed for):** by using a stethoscope, your anaesthetist can ensure that your breathing tube is not inserted too deeply and that you do not have any areas of blockage in your lungs. Other methods use a special meter to assess the size or volume of each breath you take or are given; or a gauge to measure the pressure in your lungs between breaths and the pressure that is required to inflate your lungs with each breath. The latter is known as your pulmonary inflation pressure.
- **Your nerve and muscle function:** by using a peripheral nerve stimulator to check how the muscle relaxants are affecting your muscle activity and power.
- **Your temperature:** by using a thermometer, to ensure that you don't get too hot or too cold, since you lose some of your ability to control your temperature while anaesthetised.
- **How much urine you are producing:** by inserting a catheter into your bladder during some operations and examinations. This allows your bladder to drain freely and also gives your anaesthetist an idea of how well your kidneys are functioning.
- **The pressures in your large veins and your heart:** by inserting a special cannula into a large vein in either your neck or your arm and passing the cannula through into the large blood vessel (superior *vena cava*) that leads to the heart. Sometimes the cannula is actually threaded through the chambers of

the heart and into your pulmonary artery (which carries blood
to the lungs.) As well as pressures, the cannula can determine
how much blood your heart is pumping with each beat.

- **The depth of your anaesthetic, and whether or not you
  are unconscious** (if you are having a general anaesthetic):
  by using a monitor that looks at small electrical impulses or
  'brain waves' generated by the brain. (This is similar to an
  ECG of the brain.)

This last monitor is not available in many centres. Currently
most anaesthetists do not have access to a monitor that indicates
if you are adequately anaesthetised or aware of your surroundings.
This kind of monitor is still under development. But current anaesthetic practice is different from that of, say, ten years ago, in that
your anaesthetist can now measure with an anaesthetic agent monitor exactly how much anaesthetic agent you are receiving. This
measurement tells your anaesthetist that you are receiving enough
anaesthetic gas to ensure that you are unconscious.

Your anaesthetist also constantly observes a number of measurements from the anaesthetic machine. These include:

- the pressure of oxygen and nitrous oxide in the pipelines or
  tanks on the back of the machine from which these gases are
  delivered
- the amount of oxygen flowing to you from the machine
- the number of times each minute that the breathing machine
  (or ventilator) delivers a breath to you
- the amount or concentration of anaesthetic agents in the gas
  you breathe in and out
- that you are still connected to the breathing circuit, and that
  this circuit has not become disconnected.

The last observation is vital, because you may have been given
drugs which stop you from breathing. You must remain connected
to the breathing circuit to make sure that you continue to receive
oxygen. If your breathing circuit becomes disconnected, you could
suffer brain damage or death if the disconnection is not detected
in time.

These two lists give an idea of the large number of monitors
used. Specialty societies and regulatory bodies in anaesthesia have

published guidelines describing the equipment and monitors necessary to provide anaesthetic care. Examples are:

- The Guidelines to the Practice of Anaesthesia as Recommended by the Canadian Anaesthetists' Society
- The Australian and New Zealand College of Anaesthetists Professional documents
- The Recommendations for Standards of Monitoring during Anaesthesia and Recovery, published by the Association of Anaesthetists of Great Britain and Ireland.

One function of these guidelines is to provide details of the absolute minimum type and number of monitors that should be present, functioning, and used before an anaesthetic is given. This is similar to the 'Minimum Equipment List' required in aviation before a pilot can take off.

By now you have an idea of the amount and complexity of information that your anaesthetist must constantly observe and monitor. Currently there is no 'black box' like the one used in aviation that can integrate all the measurements and provide a 'flight profile' for your anaesthetic and operation. Some new anaesthetic machines do incorporate automated record-keeping systems, which help to document and integrate some of this information. Automated systems offer advantages in that a record can be kept during emergencies when the anaesthetist may be very busy (as described later).

Another similarity to aeroplanes is that the anaesthetic machine also has self-checking and monitoring capabilities, so that problems can be easily identified. There is always a back-up system, so that if the system fails, or there is a power blackout, the anaesthetist can safely carry the patient through such a crisis. In many ways the anaesthetist is indeed like a pilot, flying the plane, watching the instruments, and looking out the window (at the surgeon), always ready to take control if a problem occurs. This concept is also emphasised in the equipment guidelines mentioned above. In addition to listing pieces of equipment, these documents also recommend that the most important monitor of the anaesthetised patient is the continuous presence of an anaesthetist.

Chapter 3

Meet your fellow patients

None of these patients wanted to have an anaesthetic. They all wanted or needed to have an operation. But to do so, they had to have some form of anaesthetic and they all had questions. Some, like John, had only a few. Others, like Matthew, wanted to understand the advantages and disadvantages of various anaesthetic options in considerable detail. Here are their stories.

JOHN

John is a 60-year-old mechanic who has smoked a packet of cigarettes daily since he was about 16. He is also partial to a couple of beers each night after work. Last year he developed a cough, and then two months ago his *sputum* changed from whitish to rusty-coloured. His wife, Mary, persuaded him to go to the doctor, who promptly ordered a chest X-ray. Unfortunately this showed a shadow in the top of John's left lung. Because of the risk that the shadow might represent lung cancer, John's doctor then referred him to a chest surgeon. He advised John that he needed to undergo an examination of the lungs by *bronchoscopy* and also of the space in front of the heart inside the chest by *mediastinoscopy*. During these examinations, the surgeon would take a small piece of tissue or *biopsy* to determine if there was cancer present, what type it was, and if it had spread to the *lymph nodes*.

John commented, 'The surgeon told me that if it had spread to the nodes, then there was no point in me undergoing an operation to remove the cancer, that I'd be better off having some radiation. But if we'd caught it early, then my chances were pretty good that I could have part or all of my lung removed. But I'd need to have the first biopsy operation under general anaesthesia.'

LILY

Lily is a 26-year-old woman who moved from Asia five years ago to complete her education. She and her husband Tom are both university students. Having arrived in the country by different routes at about the same time, they met in one of their classes and married about two years ago.

Lily is now expecting her first baby. When she was six months pregnant, her doctor ordered a routine *ultrasound* examination of the baby. This showed no problems with the baby, but the *placenta* was positioned lower than normal in the womb. (The placenta is the organ that lines the uterus and provides the link between the mother's and the baby's circulation.) The obstetrician asked Lily to undergo a repeat examination, at seven and then at eight months. He wanted to see if the placenta had moved upwards as the baby had grown and the womb or uterus had enlarged, as can sometimes occur. If the placenta remains low, then it can block the passage of the baby through the birth canal and cause severe bleeding. For these reasons, a *Caesarean section* may be required. However, Lily had read in a magazine that the ultrasound examination might hurt the baby and so she did not go for the repeat examinations.

Lily's obstetrician has informed her of the pros and cons of attempting to deliver naturally (or a 'trial of labour') versus an elective Caesarean section. However, without the results of the ultrasound examination, the obstetrician is unable to say how safe an attempt at a natural birth might be. Tom is not sure how to react. Lily has spoken with her mother by telephone. 'My mother said I should just trust in nature. She had seven children without any problems. I really want to have my baby the normal way.'

MATTHEW

Matthew is a 37-year-old barrister who is in the middle of preparing for a large and important court case. He works long hours, eats irregularly, and has had long-standing problems with bowel function. He finally went to see a surgeon with whom he plays squash. The surgeon examined Matthew and determined that he needed to have a *haemorrhoidectomy*.

Matthew says, 'I really didn't like the idea but I couldn't go on as I was, with the pain and bleeding, particularly with this case coming up. The surgeon reassured me that I'd be out of hospital the next day and back into my office the day after.'

NICOLA

Nicola is now only three weeks old, having been born four weeks prematurely. Last week, as her mother was drying her after her bath, she noticed a small lump in Nicola's groin. Very worried, she immediately called the doctor, who told her to bring Nicola to the clinic. He diagnosed a small *hernia*. This is an outpouching of part of the bowel through the wall of the abdomen, usually found in the groin in premature babies. The hernia appears as a small soft lump. The doctor suggested that, although it wasn't troubling Nicola at the moment, it should be repaired right away. Sometimes hernias can become stuck in the abdominal wall, causing blockage of the bowel, and the lump becomes painful, swollen, and hard. In fact, both the side on which there was an obvious hernia and the other side would be repaired. The other side would be done because of the increased chance of a hernia occurring there.

Nicola's mother says, 'I didn't know what to do. The thought of handing my baby over to some strangers frightened me, although I know it's a good hospital. But you never know. I mean, you read about lots of problems in the papers, kiddies dying. They're so small and helpless. How can a baby, especially Nicola who was a premmie, cope with having an anaesthetic and an operation?'

RICHARD

Richard is an 87-year-old retiree with a bad right hip that requires a replacement. Apart from this, Richard is fit for his age. He was very active until about a year ago when his hip started to cause increasing pain and limited his movement. He has had to give up bowling, and is finding it hard to dress, in particular to bend over to get his socks on by himself. More importantly for him is that work in his beloved garden is restricted.

Richard says, 'When my wife died twenty years ago, the family was keen for me to move, but I didn't want to leave my garden. I still enjoy pottering but now I can't even bend down to pull the weeds out. And what would I do in one of those retirement villages? No, I'm better off here in my own house.'

Richard had tried several types of medication from his general practitioner, who finally suggested that a hip replacement might be the right course. Richard's last experience of surgery and anaesthesia was forty years ago, when he had an operation on his nose.

'*Polyps*,' he recalls, 'not very pleasant.'

Richard was unwilling at first to consider a hip replacement, being conscious of his age. No doubt in the back of his mind he was also thinking of his dear wife who had contracted pneumonia and died after having her gall bladder out. 'She had been her usual sprightly self when she went into hospital but never came home again.'

Richard's GP made an appointment for him to see a prominent orthopaedic surgeon. Richard had maintained his private health insurance, so he was able to avoid the public hospital waiting lists and to see the surgeon within a couple of weeks.

The orthopaedic surgeon reviewed Richard's history and examined him. 'You're incredibly fit for your age—if we could fix that right hip, we'd have you jogging in no time. Mind you, the likelihood is that you'll have trouble with the other hip within the next few years too, but at the moment it's doing fine and we shouldn't worry about it.'

The surgeon explained in detail how an artificial hip worked. He showed Richard an example and then placed it over the X-ray to demonstrate how it would fit into Richard's femur (thighbone) and sit in his hip socket.

'That all looks fine,' said Richard, 'but I'm not a young man and I'm not too sure about the anaesthetic and how I'll be after the operation.'

The surgeon, acknowledging Richard's concern, replied, 'I normally have Dr McKenzie anaesthetise my patients and I truly believe he's one of the best anaesthetists available. I can make an appointment for you to see him. He has a clinic not far from here and he's there every Friday morning.'

SUSAN

Susan is a 40-year-old schoolteacher who has suffered from heavy painful periods for the last few years and has *fibroids* of the uterus. She has wanted to have a *hysterectomy* but her doctor has cautioned against this. Now, however, Susan's last Pap test shows a few irregularities. Since receiving these new results, Susan and her doctor have discussed the various treatment options. Susan also read widely on the subject and has decided that she will have the hysterectomy.

'I'm not at all worried about the operation—it's something I've wanted to have for a while,' Susan says. 'But I am really worried about the anaesthetic. My mother's aunt died during an operation—they said she couldn't take the anaesthetic. In fact, we always talk about it whenever there's an operation on TV.'

TOBY

Toby is a ten-year-old boy who needs to have his tonsils and adenoids removed. Not only has Toby had frequent bouts of tonsillitis, with repeated absences from school, but he has also had difficulty with his breathing. This difficulty occurs at night and Toby often stops breathing for short periods. This condition is related to blockage of the upper part of the throat passage and is known as *obstructive sleep apnoea*. Although Toby's parents have spent a lot of time explaining things to him, he is not too pleased about having to have the operation.

'It's not fair,' Toby says. 'It's the start of the holidays and my friend, Ben, is having a birthday party. Now I'm going to miss it.'

Chapter 4

Different patients, different options

ANAESTHETIC CHOICES

The three types of anaesthesia are general, regional, and local. All three involve the administration of drugs to produce a change in sensation, and they are frequently used in combination.

General anaesthesia

With general anaesthesia, you may think that you are 'asleep', but it's not the same thing—it is not like normal sleep. You are actually kept in a state of carefully controlled unconsciousness by means of a mixture of potent drugs that your anaesthetist has given you. During this state you do not have any conscious control over certain functions of your body, such as breathing, swallowing, and control of temperature.

Regional anaesthesia

With regional anaesthesia, your anaesthetist injects local anaesthetic drugs through a needle that is placed close to the nerve or nerves that supply the area of the body where the surgeon will operate. Local anaesthetic drugs block the impulses of nerves temporarily, so that sensations are not carried to the brain. Before inserting the regional anaesthetic needle, the anaesthetist often applies a local anaesthetic cream to the skin or injects a small amount of local anaesthetic into the skin and tissues, so that inserting the needle is less uncomfortable.

Local anaesthesia

Local anaesthesia refers to the injection of local anaesthetic directly into the tissues, rather than near the nerves as with regional anaesthesia. Sometimes this is known as 'local freezing'. Doctors often use this technique to perform minor procedures, such as suturing (sewing) cuts.

THE CHOICE OF ANAESTHETIC

Usually, three factors influence which type of anaesthetic you are given.

- The procedure to be performed must be considered. Some procedures can only be performed under general anaesthesia. For example, a patient undergoing removal of the gall bladder, whether by means of a *laparoscopic* or keyhole technique or through a standard *incision*, needs a general anaesthetic. For other procedures it is reasonable to consider whether the operation should be carried out under local, regional, or general anaesthesia, or a combination, such as combined regional and general anaesthesia. For example, a patient undergoing an examination of the knee using a special instrument called an *arthroscope* could be offered a choice of local, regional, or general anaesthesia. A patient undergoing an open-heart operation might be offered a combination of general anaesthesia and regional anaesthesia.
- The experience, expertise and preference of the anaesthetist can vary with different techniques.
- Your own preference—whether or not you prefer to be unconscious or wish to remain as conscious and in control as possible—is a factor. Most patients prefer to be unconscious for major surgical procedures. For some procedures it is increasingly common for patients not to have a general anaesthetic—for example, Caesarean section.

It is not unusual for children to have a general anaesthetic for procedures that might be done without any form of anaesthetic in an adult—for example, MRI (magnetic resonance imaging) scanning. This is because children may not understand the explanations or be able to lie still.

What degree of choice do you have?

No matter what operation, examination, or other treatment you are to undergo, you may ask your anaesthetist if there is any choice in the anaesthetic method. You should also understand that some surgeons are more comfortable operating on patients who have received one form of anaesthetic rather than another. This most often means that the patient has a general anaesthetic.

The surgeon does not choose the type of anaesthetic you receive, unless there is no anaesthetist involved in your care. However, the surgeon may discuss the choice with you and with your anaesthetist. In the same way, your anaesthetist does not choose what operation you have or how it is carried out. Again, your anaesthetist may discuss your operation with you and your surgeon, particularly if you have special anaesthetic problems.

INFORMED CONSENT

You have every right to ask questions, to receive information, and to participate in choosing the care you will receive. Asking questions and receiving information are the basis of giving informed consent.

What does 'informed' mean?

A change in legal obligation in Canada, and more recently in Australia, means that your doctor must tell you about the risks of the anaesthetic (or operation) that are serious or *material risks*. This should be done even if these material risks are very rare. The changes in law came about to make sure that you could decide to have an anaesthetic and an operation (or other procedure) only after having weighed all the pros and cons. The discussion you have with your anaesthetist should include the possibility of a choice of anaesthetic method (if appropriate) and the risks and benefits associated with the choices. Only then should you agree or consent to undergo examination or treatment.

Having agreed to have the examination or treatment, you are then required to sign a piece of paper that describes the examination or treatment. Your signature should be dated and witnessed. This is known as giving written consent. Written consent, however, is normally obtained only for the operation or procedure for which an anaesthetic must be given. In Australia, Canada, and the United Kingdom, a separate written consent for anaesthesia is not routinely obtained. This means that written consent for the operation includes consent for the anaesthetic. Occasionally, you may be asked to give separate written informed consent for the anaesthetic. This might occur if you agreed to undergo a technique that is not routinely carried out or one that involves considerable or unusual risk.

In fact, the piece of paper that you (and all patients) sign is only that—a piece of paper—although it is a very important one in the hospital admission process. What is more important is the discussion that you have with the treating doctor before signing the form. This discussion enables you to give consent on the basis that you understand the treatment and implications to your satisfaction. The consent you give after this kind of discussion is called informed consent.

WHAT IF I DECIDE I DON'T WANT TO HAVE THE OPERATION?

If you have second thoughts, even at the last minute, you should discuss them with your surgeon and your anaesthetist. Ultimately, the decision as to whether or not to proceed with the operation is yours.

CAN I CHOOSE MY ANAESTHETIST?

It is sometimes possible to choose your anaesthetist, but there are factors which may make this difficult.

• The anaesthetist you want may not have hospital privileges, which means that the anaesthetist is not legally entitled to practise medicine in a particular institution. This does not imply any lack of skill, but rather indicates that the anaesthetist does not normally practise at that institution. (This may apply to surgeons as well.)

- Some anaesthetists and surgeons often work as a team and develop a close working relationship. A particular anaesthetist may therefore not work regularly with a particular surgeon.
- Other anaesthetists may choose to practise anaesthesia only for certain types of operations—for example, cardiac anaesthetists may not look after women undergoing labour and delivery, and paediatric anaesthetists may not provide anaesthetic care for adults.
- Although an anaesthetist may work with a particular surgeon or provide care for a patient undergoing a particular operation, the anaesthetist may not regularly use a particular type of anaesthetic—for example, regional anaesthesia.
- The anaesthetist might not be available, having been on call the night before, on holiday, or otherwise engaged.

Nevertheless, you are entitled to ask if you may have a particular anaesthetist look after you.

Chapter 5

Evaluation for your anaesthetic

Once you have agreed to have a procedure (such as an operation, an X-ray, or a special test of your stomach or bowel) you undergo two types of evaluation. The first is a general evaluation of your condition, including the problem for which you are having the operation or special test. The second is evaluation for anaesthesia.

These two types of evaluation might be carried out by a number of different individuals. They may include your family practitioner, your surgeon, your anaesthetist, another anaesthetist, another specialist doctor (such as a heart specialist or cardiologist), a dentist, or a nurse. Part of this evaluation might be carried out in the office of your general practitioner, where you might answer a questionnaire and be examined. The evaluation by your surgeon might be restricted to the specific problem for which you have seen your surgeon, for example for a *cataract*. If so, then you might be asked to see another specialist, for example a physician or *internist*, who then carries out a more general evaluation of you.

Ideally, before having an anaesthetic your surgeon or family practitioner would refer you to an anaesthetic assessment clinic. This may be because you have several health problems, such as high blood pressure, heart disease, and asthma. Or you may have an unusual condition, be taking special medications, or be booked to undergo a long or complex surgical procedure. Most importantly, you should be referred if you or any of your relatives have had problems with anaesthetics in the past. You may, however, ask to see a specialist anaesthetist if you have any of the above problems or are simply worried about having an anaesthetic.

If you are booked to undergo an anaesthetic evaluation, it is important that you attend. One of the goals of the evaluation is to minimise any foreseeable risks.

THE ANAESTHETIC ASSESSMENT CLINIC

You may be asked to attend the clinic anywhere from one day to several weeks before your planned procedure. Most clinics operate during the day, so you may have to take additional time from work or home.

The anaesthetist who sees you records the findings on an anaesthetic record or consultation sheet. This information usually becomes part of your *hospital record* or chart, along with information from your surgeon.

Which person you see in the clinic depends on the type of clinic to which you are referred. In some clinics, a specially assigned nurse may ask you certain questions. Depending on your answers, you might then be seen by an anaesthetist who is working in the clinic that day. In other clinics you will always be seen by an anaesthetist.

Whether or not you are evaluated at this time by the anaesthetist who will actually give your anaesthetic care depends on where you live. You might undergo evaluation by your anaesthetist some time before the scheduled procedure. This evaluation might be carried out in the anaesthetist's office, in a freestanding clinic, in a hospital-based clinic, or in the hospital before the procedure is undertaken. Sometimes, because of the way anaesthetics and operations are scheduled in hospitals, it is less likely that your

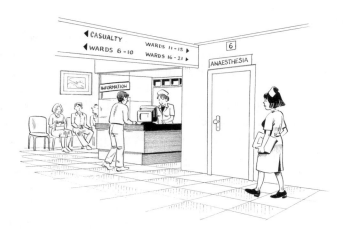

evaluation will be carried out by your particular anaesthetist. Instead, another member of the Department of Anaesthesia who is working in the clinic that day will probably evaluate you. This doctor relays the information about you to the anaesthetist who cares for you during your procedure.

If you have a number of health problems, you may also be seen in consultation by a physician or an internist, or by a specialist such as a cardiologist. The information from all these specialists is put together to provide a complete picture of any problems that you have, and any that might occur either during or after your operation.

What sort of things do they want to know?

In general, you are asked to give a complete history—your medical story. During the process of being evaluated and before undergoing your anaesthetic and procedure you might be asked the same questions more than once. Although it is tempting to assume that the information has already been recorded, it is vital that you answer the questions as fully as possible each time.

Your medical history includes details about the problem for which you are having the operation or procedure, and your current state of health. Your anaesthetist wants to know if you have any difficulties such as asthma or chronic bronchitis. If you wheeze at night, after exercise, or out in cold air, or are prone to frequent chest infections, you should tell your anaesthetist. It is also important to mention if you are using any inhalers, which one(s), and how often. Your heart function is also crucial information, particularly if you have any chest pain or angina, high blood pressure, or an irregular heartbeat. Other important conditions include diabetes, glandular problems such as thyroid disease, kidney disease, and liver disease. In addition, certain diseases are important in determining how an anaesthetic might be given, such as *malignant hyperthermia* (MH). (See chapter 6.)

Your past health is also of interest, including any operations you have had, and whether or not you, or any of your relatives, have had any problems with an anaesthetic. You will also be asked about allergies and any medications or tablets you are taking. Bring all the medications with you, including any herbal preparations, vitamins, and over-the-counter remedies (non-prescription drugs) that you are taking. Because it is easy to forget things, particularly details about operations in the past, it is helpful to write out a list of key events in your medical history. This is useful not only for this encounter but also for any in the future.

What sorts of things does the anaesthetist look at?

Your anaesthetist will then examine you. The three major areas that are of most importance to your anaesthetist are your *airway*, your breathing, and your circulation.

The airway is the part of the body from your mouth and nose to the bottom of your windpipe or trachea. Evaluation involves looking at several parts:

- **Your mandible or lower jaw:** The size and the shape, as well as its relation to where your voice-box or *larynx* is.
- **Mouth opening:** How widely your mouth opens and if you have any pain or clicking in your jaw when you do so.
- **Uvula:** How much of this structure (which lies at the back of your throat) can be seen when you open your mouth as widely as possible.

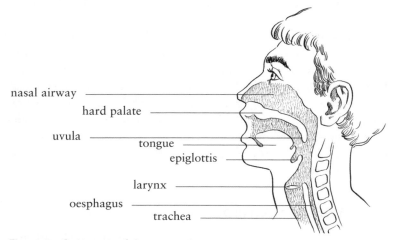

Figure 2   Structures of the upper airway.

- **Teeth:** The number, position, and condition of your teeth, and whether or not you have dentures or bridges.
- **Head movements:** How well you can bend your head forwards, backwards, and sideways.
- **Your general shape:** Whether or not you have a large stomach or large breasts, a *goitre* in your neck, or any curvature or deformity of your spine.

Careful assessment of all of these parts of your body helps your anaesthetist decide how easy it will be to take control of your airway, to ensure that your breathing does not become partially blocked or completely obstructed.

After measuring your blood pressure and heart rate, your anaesthetist usually listens to your heart and lungs with a stethoscope. Also, as part of the general evaluation, you are weighed and your height is measured. These results are of importance in helping your anaesthetist calculate the doses of drugs to give you.

Will I have to have any tests?

Depending on your age, general health, and the proposed operation, you may be asked to have some blood and urine tests, an X-ray of your chest, and an electrocardiogram (ECG or EKG). Other tests may also be ordered—for example, an X-ray of your neck if you have problems such as severe *rheumatoid arthritis*, or a *stress test* of your heart if you complain of chest pains when you are resting or walking about slowly. Your surgeon may have ordered some of these tests and your anaesthetist may add or subtract tests. If you have recently had tests, such as a check of your blood count (*haemoglobin*), or a chest X-ray, then your anaesthetist will appreciate knowing the results. It may be possible to have the results of tests forwarded to the clinic or hospital from your general practitioner or wherever the tests were carried out. This saves having to repeat the tests and helps to keep down the costs of health care.

The ASA classification

In the last part of pre-anaesthetic assessment, the anaesthetist makes an overall evaluation of you and assigns a numerical classification.

This is known as the ASA Class, where ASA stands for American Society of Anesthesiologists. Although it was developed in the United States, the ASA Class is now used worldwide as a way of classifying patients according to how well or ill they are. This classification refers only to your physical condition at the time of assessment. The higher the score, the less well you are. An 'E' after the appropriate classification designates that you are to undergo an *emergency* operation.

- **ASA Class I:** a normal healthy patient
- **ASA Class II:** a patient with mild systemic disease
- **ASA Class III:** a patient with severe systemic disease limiting activity but not incapacitating
- **ASA Class IV:** a patient with incapacitating systemic disease that is a constant threat to life
- **ASA Class V:** an extremely ill patient who is not expected to live 24 hours with or without an operation.

The ASA classification is *not* a score of how risky the anaesthetic might be for you. However, the ASA Class has been shown to correlate with the risk of complications occurring after the operation, particularly the risk of dying. This risk is related to the operation performed and how well or ill a patient was before the procedure (or a patient's preoperative physical condition). In general, there is very little contribution from the anaesthetic to the chance of a patient dying after a procedure.

Chapter 6

Preparation for your anaesthetic

Both psychological and physical preparation is important for having an anaesthetic.

PSYCHOLOGICAL PREPARATION

Psychological preparation includes providing you with education about your anaesthetic, operation, or procedure, your hospital stay and your postoperative course. Most patients want to know as much as possible about their own health care, including their role, and are no longer prepared to accept statements from doctors such as 'I know what's best'.

Children

Children are one group of patients who need special psychological preparation. The effects of hospitalisation on children are related to age; length of stay; parental factors; and the child's previous experiences of hospital or medical care. These in turn affect how long it takes to prepare a child and also what information should be given.

Age

How a child reacts to hospitalisation depends on his or her age. This, in turn, determines the length of preparation.

- **From six months to four years of age:** Small children are psychologically most vulnerable and do not understand the necessity for treatment. They recognise threatening situations but are unable to comprehend explanations or reassurances. Preparation takes from a few hours to a day.

- **From four to six years:** These children are more accepting of explanation and reassurance and need to be prepared a few days ahead.
- **From six to ten years:** These children are less likely to have a problem with separation, but there are more fears of anaesthesia, surgery, and pain. They may have fantasies of mutilation, but are amenable to reassurance, although they may become irritable or impatient. Their preparation may take a week or so.
- **Adolescents** fear loss of control and dying. They resent restricted activity and lack of privacy, and are more likely to have underlying emotional problems. As a parent you should recognise that preparation for a teenager should take at least a week.

Length of stay

The expected length of the hospital stay also determines the extent of psychological preparation. An overnight stay has a different effect from a day visit to the hospital. Children undergoing operations that might require weeks of hospitalisation need careful preparation.

Parental factors

Hospitalisation has less effect on children who are accustomed to parental substitutes and who have been subjected to less protective parenting. Children can also sense parental anxiety, and show similar signs of anxiety and stress, which may not appear until the actual start of the anaesthetic.

A child's previous experiences of hospital or medical care

The first hospital experience is the most important one and influences all subsequent visits.

What to tell your child

The most important feature of preparing children for anaesthesia and surgery is honesty. Children expect to be told the truth and lose confidence in anyone who gives them misleading information. An example is when a parent tells a child that he or she is going to hospital for a 'visit', or worse still when a parent does not tell the child that he or she is going to hospital, let alone having an operation.

The greatest fear children have in relation to hospitalisation is 'needles'. The prospect of having a needle or injection must be discussed openly. Parents and guardians must never use the threat of a needle by a doctor or nurse as a punishment.

Many things have changed in anaesthetic practice, including the giving of premedication by injection. This is now uncommon— especially for children. If some form of premedication is needed, then it is more often given in the form of a tablet or liquid. (See below.) Also, when injections do need to be given, local anaesthetic cream is commonly applied beforehand, making the process much less painful. As a parent or guardian you are entitled to ask whether or not these options are available for your child from your anaesthetist and hospital.

As well as talking with your child, there are other things that you can do to help with psychological preparation. You should take an active part in any preparation, such as reading books, watching videos, and visiting a preadmission clinic or the hospital with your child. (See Appendix 1: What you can do to help.)

Adults having major surgery

Some adults require special preoperative psychological preparation. Some operations may lead to a decrease in intellectual abilities— for example, major brain or open-heart operations. Other patients are at risk because of pre-existing medical conditions, such as age-related loss of memory. Intellectual impairment might be of short- or long-term duration and tends to increase the length of stay in hospital. Problems may range from a brief episode of postoperative confusion to complete inability to function without total care, which is extremely rare.

Your surgeon may have already discussed this with you and your family. It is also important to discuss it with your anaesthetist and with your family. As well, some thought should go to planning how to cope after your operation. Take into account the possibility of an increased length of stay in the hospital, the need for long-term care and extra care at home—from family and/or professional helpers. Some patients like to get all their affairs in order. Others wish only to make arrangements for someone to look after the garden or a pet.

PHYSICAL PREPARATION

The physical preparation includes directions to follow specific instructions about medications and fasting.

Medications

There are two types of medications which you might be asked to take before your anaesthetic. The first group is the regular medications or tablets that you are already taking. The second group is additional medications that your doctors might prescribe before your anaesthesia and operation or procedure. This second group of drugs is traditionally referred to as the 'premed'. Many people think of the 'premed' as being a tablet or injection given to produce a state of calmness. In fact, the term *premedication* refers to the ordering of all drugs before anaesthesia and surgery.

Regular medications

You may be taking several different medications, particularly if you are old, or have a chronic condition such as high blood pressure, heart disease, asthma, or diabetes. In the past, anaesthetists often asked their patients to stop taking some of these tablets before anaesthesia. However, anaesthetists now prefer that their patients continue to take almost all their medications, right up to the time of surgery.

There are three major exceptions to this recommendation.

The first is a specific class of drugs used to treat depression, known as monoamine oxidase inhibitors or MAOIs. There is a risk of a serious drug interaction between the MAOI drug and adrenaline (epinephrine) or pethidine (meperidine), producing over-excitation of the brain and a potentially fatal rise in blood pressure. (The same reaction can occur if you are taking an MAOI drug and eat mouldy cheese or drink red wine.) If you are taking this type of drug and you need to have an anaesthetic, then you and your GP or psychiatrist should arrange for the drug to be stopped before your anaesthetic. However, if you need to have an emergency operation or have not stopped taking the drug, tell your anaesthetist so he or she can avoid giving you any of the drugs which may interact.

The second exception is drugs used to thin the blood. If you are taking warfarin or coumadin, then you must check with both your anaesthetist and your surgeon for specific instructions on when and how to taper the dose of these drugs. If you have had a stroke or been threatened with one, you may be taking a type of drug known as an anti-platelet agent, or one of the non-steroidal anti-inflammatory drugs such as aspirin. You may also be taking aspirin because of heart problems or arthritis. Again, you should check with your anaesthetist and surgeon. These drugs have an effect on how certain cells in the bloodstream (platelets) stick to each other when blood clots. Because the cells are no longer so sticky, there can be more bleeding during and after operations. The effects of these drugs on blood clotting may last for as long as 14 days. Some patients can stop taking these drugs without any problems before anaesthesia and surgery. However, other patients should not stop them, including those with very bad heart disease or a past stroke. Also, patients who rely on these drugs for relief of pain and other symptoms from their arthritis may find that their joints are much more painful if they stop the tablets. Again, it is vital to ask the doctor who normally looks after you, and your anaesthetist and surgeon.

The third exception is tablets for the control of blood sugar for diabetes. If you normally take this kind of drug, you should not do so on the day you are to have your anaesthetic. If you do so and then go without eating (fast), your blood sugar might drop very low while you are under the anaesthetic and cannot complain of symptoms of low blood sugar or hypoglycemia. In addition, one of these drugs, metformin, has been associated with the development of a severe condition where acid builds up in the bloodstream.

The risk of this developing is more likely in patients who undergo certain procedures, such as heart operations where the heart-lung machine is used.

On the other hand, if you are taking insulin for control of diabetes, you will want to discuss how best to manage your insulin. Ideally, patients with diabetes should be scheduled to undergo their procedures as the first case of the day. This allows them more time during the day to recover and perhaps to start back on a reasonably normal diet. Some diabetics are asked to take less than their normal dose of insulin. A few diabetics might even omit taking any insulin until the procedure is over and they are capable of eating or drinking again. All diabetic patients should have their blood sugar tested immediately before the operation and again when they arrive in the Recovery Room. Some patients also have their blood sugar tested during the procedure by their anaesthetist.

I'm taking tablets. Is this important?

Telling your anaesthetist exactly what tablets and medications you are taking is one of the most important things you can do. This includes both prescription and non-prescription drugs, including alcohol and nicotine. You should also mention if you are taking any herbal preparations and vitamins. Some of these may interact with anaesthetic drugs, as well as those used to relieve pain in the postoperative period. For example, St John's Wort is a herbal preparation commonly used by patients who are feeling 'blue' or a little depressed. This herb is known to affect the length of time that certain prescription drugs last.

Other non-prescription items of importance are antacids, such as Mylanta, Maalox, or Pepto-Bismul. These antacids come either as a thick creamy liquid or as tablets. You should not take any of these after the midnight before your operation. If inhaled into your lungs, these antacids can cause damage from the tiny particles from which they are made.

I've used street drugs in the past. Should I tell my anaesthetist?

It is vital for your anaesthetist to know what drugs you have used in the past and when. Street or 'recreational' drugs, such as heroin,

LSD, and cocaine, can strongly influence the anaesthetic. Cocaine and ecstasy are two drugs that excite the nervous system. They may excite your heart, producing dangerous swings in blood pressure and heart rate, both during and after the operation. Drugs such as LSD can produce hallucinations, which may cause flashbacks in the postoperative period. As a general rule, it is safer not to use any of these drugs for at least one week before your anaesthetic and operation.

Is it true that I shouldn't go to the pub the night before my operation?

Yes, anaesthetists recommend that you do not have anything alcoholic to drink on the day before and the day of the operation. In general, patients who drink alcohol every day need higher doses of anaesthetic drugs than those patients who do not consume any alcohol. So it is also important to tell your anaesthetist exactly how much alcohol you drink and how often.

When should I stop smoking?

Ideally, you should stop smoking six months before the operation. If you do quit, you may notice that you have a cough and are bringing up some phlegm. This is usually a sign that your lungs are starting to recover from the effects of the nicotine and the smoke. However, you may not have that much time to quit before the operation, or you may be unable to quit entirely. In either case, decreasing the number of cigarettes and the amount smoked of each cigarette will help. Using nicotine gum or a nicotine patch may make it easier, although neither should be used on the day you have your anaesthetic.

ADDITIONAL MEDICATIONS

You may also be given other drugs before the anaesthetic. These drugs may be prescribed to make you less anxious, to relieve pain, to lessen the risk of your inhaling stomach acid into your lungs, and to lessen the possibility of postoperative nausea and vomiting. In addition, you may also be given antibiotics to reduce the risk of infection. In the past many of these drugs were given by injection. However, anaesthetic practice has changed and now almost all of these drugs can be given in tablet or liquid form.

Will I be given a sedative premed before my operation?

If you are extremely anxious, ask your anaesthetist or your surgeon for something to calm you. In the past, many different drugs were used to help patients feel less anxious before anaesthesia. These drugs included barbiturates and antihistamines. Currently, you might receive one of a class of drugs known as benzodiazepines, such as midazolam, temazepam, or diazepam. You may be given a single tablet, or a prescription for something to take at home the night before the operation. Or you may be given a tablet, or less often an injection, once you arrive at the hospital. However, many patients are not admitted to hospital until shortly before the operation. Because of this, you might not receive any form of sedative premed.

Do I have to have a sedative premed?

You may prefer not to receive any form of sedation, as this will enable you to remain in control for as long as possible before your anaesthetic and operation. Another reason is that studies have shown that patients who do not receive any sedation recover from the effects of the anaesthetic more quickly than those who were sedated beforehand. Older patients tend to remain sleepy for longer and may also have some problems with memory when sedated to reduce preoperative anxiety.

Drugs to relieve pain

In the past, patients were often given an injection of a narcotic, such as pethidine. This injection was designed to help reduce anxiety and also to supplement the drugs given at the time of the anaesthetic. Many anaesthetists no longer give pain-relieving drugs until the patient is actually in the Operating Room, unless the patient is already in pain. Some patients, such as those undergoing open-heart surgery, may be given an injection of a sedative and a narcotic. This helps to ensure that they are calm before the operation and that the heart is not stressed.

I'm taking pain tablets—should I stop them?

If you are taking painkillers, such as narcotics, it is important to continue taking them so that your pain does not get out of control. But your anaesthetist needs to know about them in order to plan which drugs to give you both during and after the operation. (See also 'Relief of postoperative pain' in chapter 8.)

Drugs to lessen the risk of inhaling stomach acid into the lungs

Another group of drugs that you might be given are those that lessen your risk of inhaling some of the acid contents of your stomach into your lungs, either during or after anaesthesia. If you are so unfortunate as to suffer this complication, there is an immediate risk of suffocation by any large pieces of partially digested food that are present in your stomach. There is also a later risk of severe pneumonia from the acid contacting delicate lung tissue. This complication is known as pulmonary *aspiration* of gastric acid and is potentially lethal.

Three types of drugs can be used to lessen the chances of this occurring in patients who are considered at risk:

- **A drug that decreases the production of acid:** This type of drug is known as a histamine-2 (H-2) receptor-blocking agent, such as cimetidine or ranitidine.
- **Sodium citrate to take by mouth:** Sodium citrate is an antacid and makes your stomach contents less acid (by increasing the pH level). Unlike other antacids, sodium citrate is a clear liquid and does not contain any small particles that could damage your lungs if you inhale any stomach contents.

- **A drug to increase the rate at which your stomach empties into the small intestine,** thus decreasing the volume of fluid in your stomach. One drug used for this purpose is metoclopramide.

There are no set rules or strict guidelines for the use of any of these drugs. If you were to undergo a Caesarean section, you might be given some sodium citrate. Some anaesthetists use H-2 receptor blockers in patients who have a *hiatus hernia* or heartburn. If you are extremely obese (fat), you might be given all three types of drugs. (People who are very fat tend to have large volumes of very acid fluid in the stomach.)

If you have suffered from nausea and vomiting after a previous procedure, you might be given an anti-emetic. Droperidol is frequently given through the intravenous line at the start of the anaesthetic. If you are given this drug by injection into the muscle (intramuscularly) some hours preoperatively, there is a chance that you might experience an unpleasant psychological reaction known as *dysphoria*. (This is the opposite of *euphoria*.) Other drugs that are used to prevent nausea and vomiting include scopolamine (which may be given by a patch placed on the skin), Stemetil and Gravol. A recently introduced group of drugs is extremely effective in preventing postoperative nausea and vomiting, although they are very expensive. One example of this group is ondansetron, which may be taken in tablet form or injected intravenously. If not given preoperatively, many anti-emetics may be given during the operation.

Drugs to reduce infection

In addition, your surgeon may ask that you be given a dose of antibiotics before the procedure. This is most likely if you are to undergo an operation on your bowel, bladder, or reproductive organs. Your surgeon may also order antibiotics if you are having a device, such as a pacemaker, implanted. Generally, your anaesthetist is not responsible for ordering antibiotics for this purpose, although he or she might order 'prophylactic' antibiotics if you have problems with your heart valves. (Another doctor, such as a heart specialist or surgeon, may also take responsibility for ordering them.)

Sometimes these antibiotics are given in the hour before the operation. In other cases your anaesthetist administers them, usually at the start of the anaesthetic. This ensures that the amount of antibiotic in your blood is as high as possible at the time of the operation.

WHEN WILL I BE ADMITTED TO THE HOSPITAL?

If you had an operation in the past, then chances are that you were admitted to hospital one to two days beforehand. During this period you underwent all the steps necessary for preparation for anaesthesia and surgery, being examined by various doctors, undergoing tests, and meeting with your anaesthetist the evening before surgery.

Now, in many parts of the English-speaking world, patients are no longer admitted to hospital the night before the operation. Instead, they are admitted on the day of the procedure for all elective surgery. This is known by such terms as 'Admit Day of Procedure' (ADOP) or 'Day of Surgery Admission'. Patients arrive at the hospital for admission as little as one to two hours before the operation. This shortened period of hospital stay is more efficient, allowing more patients to be treated in a hospital than previously.

How will the doctors know that there's nothing else wrong with me?

Because you probably will not be admitted to the hospital until a few hours before the operation, all the tests and preparation that would once have been done when you were in the hospital are done in the days or weeks before. You may be asked to attend an anaesthetic assessment clinic or preadmission clinic, where you will be evaluated (see chapter 5).

What happens if I need an emergency operation?

If you require an emergency operation, your anaesthetist needs to assess you quickly. If time permits, you are assessed in the Accident and Emergency Unit or on the ward; otherwise the assessment takes place when you arrive in the Operating Room. In life-threatening emergencies, the opportunity for your anaesthetist to assess you is obviously very limited. Often your anaesthetist only has the opportunity to ask you a few specific questions, such as 'Do you have any allergies?', 'Do you take any medication?', 'Have you had any problems with anaesthetics in the past?' These questions might be asked as your anaesthetist starts intravenous lines and attaches monitors. Frequently, your anaesthetist must rely on your surgeon and other doctors or paramedical staff to provide an overall summary of your previous health and your current condition. In addition, anaesthetists rely on their own observational skills. In extreme emergencies, there may be no opportunity for your anaesthetist to discuss with you the options or risks of anaesthetic care. However, it is still routine practice for your anaesthetist to assess and document your ASA Classification (see chapter 5).

WHY IS FASTING IMPORTANT?

If you vomit when you are awake, or even when you are asleep at night (and not anaesthetised), your reflexes prevent any of that vomit being sucked into your lungs. You cough and splutter to clear the area around the back of your throat and larynx. Then you can breathe again.

When anaesthetised (or very drunk, or affected by an overdose of sedatives or certain street drugs), you may be able to vomit but some of your protective reflexes do not work. There is therefore a risk that fluid from the stomach will regurgitate—that is, run up your oesophagus and into the back of your throat. Should this happen when your level of consciousness is decreased, you cannot protect yourself by swallowing and coughing. The fluid may then pass into your windpipe or trachea and down into your lungs. This is known as aspiration.

Should you inhale some stomach contents, there is the risk of suffocation, particularly if undigested food is present. The acid in your lungs may also cause severe wheezing and a lack of oxygen. Later, pneumonia may develop. This pneumonia is a particularly severe form because of the effect of the acid on the delicate tissue of the lungs.

When can I eat and drink?

Until about ten years ago, it was common for patients scheduled for elective surgery to fast from midnight on the night before surgery. If the operation was scheduled in the afternoon, patients had to fast for periods of up to 16–18 hours. In the late 1980s, a number of scientific studies were carried out that questioned the validity of this fasting policy. In some countries, professional organisations have changed their recommendations to allow shorter hours of fasting. For example, the Canadian Anaesthetists' Society produced a revision to the *Guidelines to the Practice of Anaesthesia* in 1996. These new guidelines stated that fasting policies should take into account the age of the patient, as well as any medical problems that the patient might have. The guidelines also recommended that a patient should not eat any solid foods on the day of surgery, but could drink clear fluids up to three hours before the operation.

Despite increasing amounts of scientific evidence about the safety of following guidelines such as these, standard textbooks of anaesthesia still recommend that patients be '*NPO*' ('Nil per os' or 'nothing by mouth') for six to eight hours before anaesthesia and surgery. It is likely that such statements will change in the future, although anaesthetists still recommend in general that patients do not eat any solid food after midnight before the scheduled operation.

Fasting in children

The situation is different with children. Infants, especially, do not tolerate long periods of fasting or restriction of fluids, which might quickly lead to dehydration. It is usual to try to minimise the fasting time for children for food or milk to six hours before the operation. Cow's milk or formula is not emptied quickly from the stomach and is considered to be similar to solid food. Breast milk, on the other hand, is emptied from the stomach more readily and a shorter fasting time is more appropriate. The length of time is often determined by the usual feeding pattern of the infant. Children may drink clear fluids up to two hours before the time of the operation. Parents should consult with the anaesthetist for advice in individual cases.

Emergency surgery

If you have been in an accident, are in pain, or have been given an injection of a painkiller, the speed at which food leaves your stomach and passes downwards is slowed. This results in you having what anaesthetists term a *full stomach*, which increases the risk of stomach contents being regurgitated back up the throat. Theoretically, your operation could be delayed until your stomach has emptied, although this is not always appropriate. There are ways of minimising the risk of *regurgitation* of gastric contents. Some patients may need to have a *nasogastric tube* inserted through the nose, down the oesophagus, and into the stomach. The fluid in the stomach can then be suctioned out through the tube, although removing solids is still a problem. This technique is important in patients who have an obstruction of the bowel. Unfortunately, suctioning cannot ensure that the stomach is empty, but only that it is 'less full'. Drugs that are currently used to lessen the risk of regurgitation include those to neutralise stomach acid, those to decrease acid production, and those to increase the downward emptying of the stomach. (See above.)

Can I keep my dentures in?

In general, you are advised to leave your dentures in safekeeping with a relative or nurse while you have your anaesthetic and operation. If your dentures become dislodged, there is a risk of interference with your anaesthetist's ability to clear your airway or to pass an endotracheal tube into your voice-box (larynx). If you are having an operation or procedure on your nose, mouth, or lung passages, then your surgeon may wish you to remove your dentures. There is also a risk that your dentures might be dropped (and broken) or lost, if they are removed while you are unconscious in the Operating Room.

Occasionally anaesthetists ask their patients to leave their dentures in, especially if they are a firm fit. It may be easier for your anaesthetist to maintain your airway with your dentures in place. Also, if you are having your procedure done under regional block or monitored anaesthesia care, you may be able to keep your dentures in. However, whether or not you do so depends on your anaesthetist.

WHAT IF I'M NOT WELL WHEN I'M SUPPOSED TO HAVE MY OPERATION?

In general, you should be as well as possible before undergoing any anaesthetic or surgery. Sometimes, of course, surgery is necessary and there may even be some degree of urgency to have the operation. In most cases, an optimal time is suggested. Your surgeon, perhaps together with your anaesthetist, can weigh up your need for the operation and how urgent it is against any illness or condition you have. One of the benefits of the developments in anaesthetic drugs and techniques is that anaesthesia is now relatively safe, even in patients who are severely ill.

What if I've got a cold or something like diarrhoea?

If you are scheduled for elective surgery, it is usual to delay the operation if you become unwell. The final decision as to whether or not to delay your operation rests with your anaesthetist and your surgeon. It is best to contact them if you become unwell in the days leading up to your appointment. You may also wish to contact your family doctor for advice and possible treatment.

If you have a cold or the flu, it is likely that your anaesthetic and operation will be postponed. If you have a sore throat with no other symptoms, your anaesthetist may consider that you can proceed, although your throat may be very sore afterwards. If the sore throat is an early sign of the development of a cold or the flu (and it isn't always), the resulting illness may be hastened and you may feel extremely unwell after the operation. Again, the decision to proceed rests with your anaesthetist and your surgeon, although if you decide not to proceed your wishes will be respected.

There is an increased risk of respiratory complications when anaesthesia is administered to a patient with an established cold or influenza. Your anaesthetist, however, is aware of the potential for complications and of the means of managing them safely.

Diarrhoea is not a contraindication to anaesthesia or surgery unless it is part of a more generalised illness.

My child is due to have her tonsils out and is never without a cold. What do we do?

Children are particularly prone to repeated colds, especially if they have problems with their tonsils or adenoids. It is not uncommon for children with chronic tonsillitis, who require tonsillectomy, to have constant symptoms of a respiratory infection. It is therefore normal to proceed with the anaesthetic and surgery in the presence of such symptoms. Ideally, one should choose a time when the child is 'relatively well'.

If the child is coughing up phlegm, has a high fever, or is lethargic (looking ill, tending to sleep, and refusing food), the operation will most likely be postponed. The period of delay of the operation may be up to six weeks, as studies have shown that the airway remains sensitive. The child is more prone to coughing and gagging and is more likely to develop some swelling in the throat during this period after a cold or the flu.

ARE THERE AGE LIMITS FOR HAVING AN ANAESTHETIC?

There are no age limits for having an anaesthetic. For example, it is now possible to anaesthetise tiny premature babies for prolonged and major operations. Nor is there any reason why elderly patients should not undergo necessary operations. Developments in drugs, equipment and techniques have made anaesthesia possible and safe for patients of all ages.

HOW SOON CAN I HAVE ANOTHER ANAESTHETIC?

There is really no minimum period when it is dangerous to have a second anaesthetic. The factors that determine if you have a second anaesthetic (or more) soon after the first one include the need for surgery, how well you recover, and what drugs are used.

With some older anaesthetics, elimination from all the body tissues took some time and small amounts stayed for several days.

This meant that doses had to be modified when a second anaesthetic was administered. Also, with an inhalational agent called halothane, there is evidence that, very rarely, a repeated anaesthetic in a short time may give rise to a higher chance of liver damage. (See below.) In children, this complication is exceedingly rare.

There are some patients who have needed repeated anaesthetics over many years. Some patients have had more than a hundred. No particular problems have been reported.

CAN MY CHILD HAVE HIS VACCINATION WHILE HE IS UNDER THE ANAESTHETIC?

If a routine vaccination by injection is due, there does not appear to be any reason why it cannot be given by the anaesthetist during your child's anaesthetic. You should discuss the matter with the anaesthetist during the preanaesthetic consultation.

WILL I NEED A BLOOD TRANSFUSION? IS IT SAFE?

The need for a transfusion of blood during surgery depends on two major factors:

- **The need to replenish any blood lost during the procedure:** In some operations it is inevitable that enough blood will be lost to require replacement. These operations include heart surgery, major orthopaedic surgery, and some abdominal surgery. In other cases there is only a possibility that blood will need to be replaced, but a supply is prepared in case. This is called 'cross-matching'.
- **The patient's preoperative blood count (or haemoglobin level):** If this is too low, then there is an increased chance of having a transfusion.

Small children are more likely to need a transfusion because the amount of blood lost during the operation represents a much greater proportion of the total amount of blood in the child's body.

For example, a newborn baby has only about 300 millilitres of blood in total.

The anaesthetist has several options for dealing with the blood loss. The simplest is to replace the lost blood with donated blood. However, this is normally done only after using other intravenous fluids as a substitute, and allowing the haemoglobin level to fall until it becomes critically low. (It is the haemoglobin that carries oxygen in the blood.)

Another option is to use a device called a 'cell saver', which anaesthetists use to collect any blood lost during the operation. The blood is filtered and then returned to the patient. Thus many operations, even the major ones mentioned above, can be performed without using donated blood, although there are some risks related to having low haemoglobin levels.

In some centres, patients can arrange to have their own blood taken in advance, stored and then made available for transfusion during surgery. In some regions, but certainly not all, parents may donate blood for use in their own children.

Erythropoietin is a compound in the body that stimulates the production of red blood cells by the body. A synthetic form of erythropietin has been developed, and some patients arrange to take this drug in advance of the operation, so as to avoid having a blood transfusion.

Some patients, however, need a transfusion of blood from another person (not related to them). The risk of getting infections, either HIV or hepatitis, from blood transfusions is now extremely low because of testing, but nevertheless it is possible. There is also a risk of allergy and of complications from the transfusion of incompatible blood, but cross-matching and checking helps to reduce this risk. If you are concerned, ask your anaesthetist and surgeon to explain the relative risks in your particular case.

JOHN

Although John considers himself fit for a 60-year-old, his general practitioner had found that his blood pressure was a little high, and heard a few squeaks and wheezes, characteristic of the long-term smoker, when examining John's lungs. Because of these findings and the concern that John might have cancer of the lung,

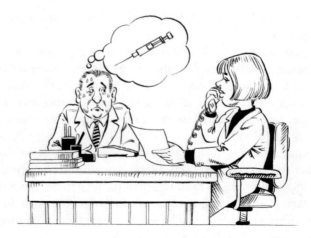

both the general practitioner and the surgeon wanted John to be evaluated further by a physician or internist.

Two weeks later, John goes to see the physician, who takes a detailed history, asking especially about John's exercise tolerance.

'Well, I reckon I'm pretty fit,' replies John, 'despite what the X-ray might show. I can still show those young blokes a thing or two. Look at these hands—they're not like that from sitting around drinking cups of tea or playing on computers.'

'How many flights of stairs can you climb?'

'Don't know, don't have any in the house.'

'What happens when you get a cold?'

'Never used to get them—but the last couple of winters, I've had some nasty bouts. Doc kept me in bed for a week last year, filled me up with antibiotics and stuff. Breathing wasn't too good then.'

'How many do you smoke in a day?'

'Oh, a packet or more.'

'How many is that?'

'Probably thirty or so.'

'That's quite a few over the years.'

The physician asks more detailed questions and then examines John, paying particular attention to his heart and lungs. He also checks John's blood pressure, looks in his eyes, and tests his reflexes. John's blood pressure is slightly high, but his heart is beating regularly and sounds normal when the physician listens to

John's chest. However, he does hear abnormal noises coming from John's lungs—a combination of crackles when John breathes in and wheezing when he breathes out.

John then undergoes some more tests, including blood tests, an electrocardiogram, breathing tests, and a *CT scan* of his chest. The blood tests show the numbers of the various blood cells, as well as some of the chemicals in the blood, such as glucose and potassium, alkaline phosphatase, and calcium. The electrocardiogram checks on how John's heart beats and if there are signs of any previous damage, such as a heart attack or *myocardial infarction* (MI). The breathing test, or pulmonary function test, assesses the size of John's lungs and how well they function—for example, the extent to which John's wheezing affects the flow of air from his lungs. The CT scan is done, of course, because of the possibility of cancer.

All of John's doctors have told him that he must stop smoking. This is not only because of the possibility of cancer but also because of the abnormal noises in John's lungs and the fact that he is going to have an anaesthetic.

The afternoon before surgery, John enters the public hospital, some 200 kilometres from home. This is so that he can undergo special treatment for his breathing. This treatment includes having a drug to dilate the passages of the lungs or *bronchi* and some physiotherapy. John arrives at the hospital at four o'clock and is soon settled into the ward. His wife, Mary, comes with him. She is very nervous about the whole thing but doesn't dare say so.

On admission, the nurse checks John's blood pressure, pulse, and temperature. Then the surgical resident is called to admit him.

At half past five, Dr Williams, the anaesthetist, comes to visit John. Dr Williams will be caring for John tomorrow morning when the surgeon performs the bronchoscopy and mediastinoscopy. In his hand, Dr Williams has a binder—John's hospital record or chart. Included in this record are the results of the tests, plus copies of the letters from John's general practitioner and the surgeon.

After introducing himself to John and Mary, Dr Williams asks John, 'Have you ever had an operation before?'

'I had my tonsils out when I was—oh, seven or eight. Can't remember much about it but I do remember a terrible smell—and being bloody sick after. Don't think I've had any others—what do you say, Mary?'

'No, dear,' Mary says.

'Fortunately things have changed a bit since then,' says Dr Williams. 'You probably had ether and it was terrible stuff. We don't use it any more, we've got much better drugs these days. Tell me, what's your general health like?'

'Oh, pretty good,' replies John.

'And you've obviously smoked a bit,' comments Dr Williams, looking at the nicotine stains on John's fingers. 'Have you managed to stop?'

'I've tried, but after forty years I'm finding it a bit difficult. Reckon I should have given up years ago, but you know what it's like. Been smoking since I was sixteen. I've been pretty good though—I've only had two or three over the last couple of days. But the worst of it is I've been coughing up a bit more phlegm.'

'That's good, it means that your lungs are starting to work properly. I'll have a listen to your chest now, and then go and look at your chest X-ray. We're going to get the physiotherapist to see you this evening and you'll also be having some special medication that the nurses will give you to help your breathing and maybe again in the morning. We want to see if we can't clear out a bit of that phlegm that's sitting in the bottom of your lungs. With chronic smoking it tends to stay there but sometimes it can cause a few breathing problems during and after the anaesthetic.'

'Is that serious?' asks John, looking a bit worried for the first time.

'Well, it doesn't make things easy but I'm quite happy that I can deal with it safely. You might find, though, that your cough will be a bit worse after the operation and you may see a little blood in your sputum. That will be from where the surgeon took the biopsy in your lungs. And about your blood pressure,' says Dr Williams, 'I see that it's up a bit. Have you been taking the tablets the physician prescribed for you?'

'Yes, Mary's made sure of that. Today the nurse said it was 160 or something. What does that mean?'

'Well, that number may not mean anything. Blood pressure does go up a bit as we get older and it may be that you were a bit tense when you were having it measured. But blood pressure has two numbers. The top number is called the systolic and measures how hard your heart is beating. The second number reflects how well your blood vessels relax between heartbeats and is called the diastolic. In your case, the second number is 90, which won't need any extra treatment before the operation. But it's something that I'll be keeping a close eye on during the operation. All the other blood tests are okay, including the various chemicals, such as your creatinine, which is a measure of kidney function. That sometimes can go up with high blood pressure. Now, I'd like to have a look at you—listen to your chest and so forth.'

Dr Williams first feels John's pulse at the wrist, looks at John's head and neck, and asks John to open his mouth and bend his neck forward and backward and turn his head sideways. He then taps the back of John's chest, listening to the hollow, drum-like sounds. Then he takes out his stethoscope and listens all over John's chest, to his heart and lungs.

'Tomorrow's operation is a bronchoscopy, where the surgeon is going to pass a long tube down your trachea or windpipe. I need to look after your breathing during the whole operation. I'll start by giving you an injection in the vein in your arm. I'll also be using some local anaesthetic on your throat.'

John replies quickly, 'No way I'm being awake for this. I want to be good and out.'

'That's not what I meant. You will be totally unconscious, but the local anaesthetic is so that you won't have a really sore throat afterwards. And you actually are having two procedures tomorrow—there's also the mediastinoscopy for which you will need a general anaesthetic.'

'Is there any danger to his lungs with the general anaesthetic, Doctor?' asks Mary. 'I've read in a magazine that people with breathing problems should only have spinals.'

'Well, sometimes we do give spinals to patients with lung problems, but not for these two procedures. That's because we would have to make you numb up to your chin. And then you wouldn't breathe very well. The other things I want to explain to you are what I'll be doing and the positions you'll be in for the procedure.'

'Positions?' asks John with a wry grin.

'For the first procedure, the bronchoscopy, you'll be lying on your back with your head on a very small pillow. Once you're anaesthetised and I've put the breathing tube in your throat, the surgeon will put the bronchoscope down through the breathing tube and see if he can get a sample of tissue. After he's done that, he'll take the bronchoscope out. He and I will then put a cushion under your shoulders, so your head will lean back more onto the pillow and the lower part of your neck will be clear of your chin.' Dr Williams proceeds to demonstrate. 'This helps the surgeon carry out the second procedure, the mediastinoscopy. But this position means that you might be a bit stiff and sore the next day. You probably don't lie around the house doing this.'

'I'll say,' says John in an amazed tone. 'I didn't realise all of this went on.'

'And while the surgeon is working, I'll be watching over you, keeping an eye on your blood pressure, heart rate and oxygen, in particular. Now, do you have any questions, either about what I've just explained or anything else?'

John looks at Mary and then back at Dr Williams. 'No thanks, Doc, reckon I'll be right.'

'Okay. Last question from me,' says Dr Williams. 'Do you need anything to help you sleep tonight?'

'A couple of beers would be about right.'

'I'd rather you didn't,' replies Dr Williams. 'I'll leave an order for a sleeping tablet, just in case.'

'I'll probably need it more than him,' says Mary in a quiet voice from the corner where she has been sitting.

LILY

Lily has previously refused any more ultrasound tests. 'I read that they were bad for the baby.'

However, on the last prenatal visit before her due date, the obstetrician tells Lily that, without the results of a recent ultrasound scan, he cannot guarantee her safety or that of the baby if Lily goes ahead with an attempt at a vaginal delivery. After much soul-searching and discussion, Lily and Tom agree that she should have the scan, in the hope of not having a Caesarean. The results of the examination indicate that the placenta has moved upward as the baby has grown and the uterus has expanded. The obstetrician tells Lily and Tom that a normal vaginal delivery is likely to be successful but there is a small risk of needing a Caesarean section. This would happen if there was additional bleeding during labour or signs of distress in the baby.

'You can go home, but we'd like you to come back right away, as soon as you go into labour. Forget what your mother said about staying home and washing the floors to strengthen the contractions.'

Turning to Tom, the obstetrician adds, 'I'm counting on you to bring her in right away—we'd like to keep a close eye on her during all of her labour.'

Tom looks at Lily and then back at the obstetrician. 'Yes, I will do that.'

'But before then, there is one other thing. I'd like an anaesthetist to see you—to talk about the anaesthetic—just in case you need a Caesarean.'

The next day, Lily goes to the hospital labour ward where she checks in, saying that she is there to see the anaesthetist. After about twenty minutes, Dr Jenkins arrives. She introduces herself, apologises for being late—'Twins,' she says—and explains that she will talk with Lily and Tom about anaesthesia for a Caesarean section.

Lily is a little unnerved by all of this and recalls her mother's words of caution. 'Would I really need an anaesthetic to have my baby?' she asks.

'Well, you don't have to have an anaesthetic if the baby arrives normally, although many women prefer the pain relief provided by an epidural. In your situation, however, I understand from your obstetrician that there is still a risk that you might need a Caesarean section, which means that you'll need to have an anaesthetic of some sort. So my job is to explain something about an epidural, because you can have one both for a normal birth and if you need a Caesarean section.'

Dr Jenkins proceeds to explain about epidurals, how the needle is inserted into the back, followed by threading in a fine plastic tube and pumping long-acting local anaesthetic into the area around the nerves as they branch off the spinal cord.

'Wouldn't I need to be asleep for the Caesarean section?'

'Not necessarily. In the past we used to use general anaesthesia, where you are totally asleep, for all Caesarean sections. Sometimes we still need to give a general anaesthetic but most of the time we use an epidural or a spinal. You don't feel any pain, and you can see and hold your baby as soon as it's born.'

'Would I have to watch the operation—the surgeon cutting me open?'

'Heavens, no. We put up a screen so you don't see anything until your baby is out and cries.'

'So why would I need an epidural for a natural birth, if I'm not having an operation?'

'Once again, it is for your comfort. It is to make sure you go through the whole thing with no pain. It makes you numb from the waist down.'

'But then I won't know when my baby is born?' cries Lily.

'You won't be completely numb,' answers Dr Jenkins. 'We can carefully control the amount of anaesthetic given so that you can get the sensation of needing to push, and you may even be able to walk around the ward when you're in labour.' After a pause Dr Jenkins continues, 'I take it that you didn't go to any prenatal classes.'

'No,' answers Lily, 'I was too busy studying for my course.'

'What we try to achieve with an epidural is the best of everything—no change in the birth process, no effect on the baby, and your being able to retain your sensation of the birth without the intense pain. We can also do the same thing with a newer technique called a combined spinal/epidural (CSE). In addition to having an epidural, we inject a small amount of anaesthetic into the fluid that surrounds your spinal cord. This technique gives much better preservation of muscle power—you can walk and even squat, but without any pain.'

'Do I get a say?'

'Why yes, of course you do, and you need to be entirely comfortable with any plans for your care. Right now I have to go and check on another patient in labour. I've brought you our pamphlet which explains your options. Why don't you two have a look at this and work out what you prefer.'

Dr Jenkins hands Lily a small pamphlet describing the pain relief options for childbirth.

'I'll be back to answer any questions you might have—probably in about twenty minutes—that's if you can wait.'

'We'll wait,' says Lily.

MATTHEW

Matthew is due to have his operation at eleven o'clock. He has been told to be at the hospital at seven, but decides that he should call at the office beforehand. He therefore arrives at a quarter past nine. 'Still plenty of time before 11 a.m.,' he thinks.

'Where have you been?' asks the ward sister, when Matthew arrives from Admission half an hour later.

'I'm not sure that's any of your business,' replies Matthew. 'My operation is not until eleven, there's over an hour to go.'

'Well, it's just that there are a lot of things to do to make sure everything is organised. We began to think that you had cancelled. Your anaesthetist was here at half-past seven to see you and now he's in the middle of the operating list.'

'Couldn't he come up after he's put the other patient to sleep?'

'He stays with each patient until the operation is finished and the patient is in the Recovery Room. He'll obviously need to tell you quite a bit about anaesthesia.'

'Is that how they justify their huge bills—sitting down and reading the paper while the surgeon does all the work?'

'No—I mean, what they charge is their affair, but the anaesthetist is certainly not reading the paper during the operation. It's their job to watch you and everything about you. Your life depends on your anaesthetist.'

'Oh well, what now, where do I go? Let's get it over with.'

The nurse shows Matthew to his room—a single room with en suite. Matthew doesn't have health insurance but is prepared to pay for private care rather than wait in a public hospital queue and share a room with others. She instructs Matthew on the use of the electronic bed, television set, sound system, and call button. She then directs him to get undressed and to put on a hospital gown.

Matthew is impatient but takes note. 'The operation will be at eleven, won't it?'

'That's when it's scheduled, but it may not be on the dot of eleven. It depends very much on how the previous operations go, whether there are any complications, and so on. Patients are not like Swiss trains, you know!'

Matthew grunts acknowledgment. He puts on the hospital gown and his own dressing gown over it, and opens his briefcase to retrieve a folder of papers.

Not long after, Dr Allen, the anaesthetist, knocks and enters the room.

'Hello, I'm John Allen, your anaesthetist,' he says, extending his hand. 'You must be Matthew.'

'That's right—who's looking after your patient?'

'Excuse me?' enquires Dr Allen.

'I thought you were busy in the Operating Room—at least that's what the nurse said.'

'Oh, we finished a little sooner than expected, so I popped up to see you while the surgeon dictates some notes.'

'He's very busy, I understand he's the best in the business. I've seen him at the club a couple of times. He's never there at lunch, though.'

'Yes, he's very good,' replies Dr Allen. 'Now, about your anaesthetic.'

'Just a quick injection and it should all be over—I'm preparing for a major brief for next week and I need to be on the ball again this afternoon,' says Matthew rather brusquely.

In a patient tone Dr Allen replies, 'It's not quite that simple. You're likely to be in a lot of pain after this operation. So one way we could manage that is with a spinal anaesthetic—which wouldn't make you sleepy afterwards.'

'I don't fancy a spinal,' responds Matthew. 'I remember one of the senior partners had a case of paralysis after a spinal anaesthetic.'

'How long ago was that?'

'Oh, not really sure, maybe fifteen, twenty years ago. That partner has pretty well retired, just comes in for a drink and a chat now and again. Still got him on the books though, QC and all, looks good for the company. But he always likes to talk about the case—how he tore into the anaesthetist on the stand.'

'Yes, I'm sure he recounts the story well,' says Dr Allen rather dryly. 'There have been a very small number of cases of paralysis or permanent nerve damage after spinal anaesthesia. But they have been exceedingly rare—although more often talked about. Nevertheless, it is a major complication which has to be considered, although the risk of major nerve damage after spinal anaesthesia is about the same as the risk of brain damage after general anaesthesia—extremely rare.'

'Well, what about a general anaesthetic—don't they wear off quickly these days?'

'Yes, they certainly wear off more quickly than they used to, but even with the shortest-acting drugs there is some hangover effect and there's also the hangover effect of any narcotics given for pain relief in the Recovery Room. You probably wouldn't be able to concentrate fully for a day or two. Whatever the case, after a haemorrhoidectomy, you'll need to be taking something for pain for the next few days and that will affect your mental function a little.'

Momentarily lost for words, Matthew reaches over and snaps his briefcase shut and then looks back to Dr Allen.

'Well, I suppose I don't have much choice, what with this case next week, and then I'm heading overseas for three weeks for some R & R. I want it fixed up before that.'

'My recommendation is for you to have a spinal. I've personally never had any complications and have probably done a couple of thousand, although I cannot promise that a complication will not occur. I can only do my best. But spinals work very well and I can do two things to try to help your particular situation. First, I'll add some narcotic to the local anaesthetic mixture. That should give you some better pain relief. Might even work for 24 hours. And second, I won't give you any sedation in the Operating Room, unless I think that you're getting too distressed. But then, you'll have to put up with the noise and the clatter, plus having your legs up in stirrups for forty minutes or so. You won't be able to see anything, though, as I'll put up a screen.'

Matthew wrinkles his nose and looks thoughtful, but says nothing.

'Now, I'll need to start an intravenous—you're right-handed, aren't you?'

'Yes, yes I am.'

'I'll put the intravenous into your left arm so you'll be able to use a pen when you get back here to your room. But if I end up giving you some sedation, then I recommend that you don't work— these are powerful drugs and I would hate you to send someone to jail because you couldn't concentrate on your paperwork.'

In response, Matthew lifts an eyebrow. 'Any other complications I should know about?'

'The other major complications include areas of numbness or changed sensation that might rarely occur if the needle hits and damages a small nerve near the spinal cord. That's not likely to happen, as you'll be awake when I put the needle in. If it touches a nerve, you'll be able to tell straight away.'

'Does that hurt?'

'It's not so much pain as the sensation you get when you hit your funny bone.'

'Anything else?' asks Matthew.

'Apart from that, there have been reports of *toxicity* to the nerves from certain local anaesthetic agents, but I don't use any of those. In addition, there is always the risk of infection that could lead to meningitis. However, I'll be using full sterile technique. All the equipment is single-use, disposable, and I've never seen it happen. You could also get *phlebitis*, or inflammation from the intravenous, but it won't be in long, and again I'll be using sterile technique to start it. Of course, you also have to recognise the possibility of complications from the operation, which, no doubt, your surgeon has fully explained to you.'

'Er,' responds Matthew, now visibly paler, 'perhaps you could just remind me of them.'

'The general surgical complications include bleeding, infection, and failure of the operation to relieve the problem. Then there are the complications from the positioning for the operation. In your case, you'll be in stirrups, with your legs bent at the hips. So there's always a risk of blood clots in the legs and nerve damage. The first is unlikely as you'll be up and about fairly soon. The nerve damage is something we all take particular care to prevent by padding all the possible pressure areas. This includes not just your legs but also your arms. Do you ever wake up in the morning with a numb arm or fingers?'

'Why yes, sometimes this left arm is just like a piece of wood, then it hurts like the devil when the sensation returns.'

'That means that you're more likely to develop nerve compression damage than someone who doesn't get this. So we'll pad you well. But it's another reason to remain awake—that way, if your arms are a bit uncomfortable, you can wiggle them about.'

'What if the spinal doesn't work?'

'There's always general anaesthesia to fall back on, if we need to proceed with the operation.'

'And what are the complications of general anaesthesia?'

'If we take the serious risks first, either death or permanent brain damage.'

'That's not very encouraging—I thought you anaesthetists were supposed to be looking after patients during the operation.'

'We are, and I will be, from the beginning until after the operation, when I'm absolutely satisfied that you are safely recovering from the anaesthetic.'

'So how could I die, then?'

'From the anaesthetic—only if you had an unforeseen reaction, say to a drug, and we couldn't save you, or if you had a heart attack during or after the operation. Of course, there's also the risk of the surgeon puncturing a large blood vessel and your haemorrhaging.'

'A heart attack? Why should I have a heart attack?'

'Heart attacks occasionally occur in young people in stressful situations without warning. But remember, I'm talking extremely rare occurrences here. From what I can tell about you—from what I've read in the notes and looking at you now—there's no reason to suggest that it would occur. I'm simply giving you full information about serious but very rare complications, so that you can make a choice.'

'What about drug reactions—you mean allergies? Wouldn't I know I was allergic to something?'

'There are two kinds of reactions. The more common one is allergy, and no, you wouldn't necessarily know that you were allergic to any of the anaesthetic agents. Sometimes the reaction can occur out of the blue. The other kind of reaction is related to a genetic predisposition. The most serious condition is called malignant hyperthermia. A very, very few families carry a gene that predisposes the patient to react to two particular types of anaesthetic agents. If those patients react, their muscles stiffen and they develop a very high fever. Without a special drug treatment, they have a 50 per cent chance of dying. But it's so rare that we've never seen a case in this hospital, and we give about 20,000 anaesthetics each year.' Dr Allen continues, 'Now, you do need to realise that I know how to recognise and treat all of these complications. It's part of anaesthetic training and we keep up-to-date, learning about new reactions and new treatments.'

'That's quite reassuring,' admits Matthew.

Just then, the nurse enters the room.

'They're calling for you in the Operating Room. Do you want to walk down with Dr Allen and me? They must be running a little late—it's 11:20.'

'Now are you comfortable with all I've told you? Is there anything else you wish to know?' asks Dr Allen.

'Yes, I'm comfortable. No, I don't want to ask anything. Let's just get on with it.'

NICOLA

Nicola and her mother arrive at the hospital at seven o'clock. The operation is scheduled for eight o'clock. Nicola is first, as it is usual to try to operate on the youngest (or sickest) patients first, so that they don't have to go without food or drink for so long. Nicola is breast-fed and she had her last feed at three o'clock in the morning.

Nicola is admitted to the neonatal ward—the ward for babies less than four weeks old or born prematurely. This is a children's hospital, so there are lots of babies. Some are in small cots and some in clear plastic box-like cots (called isolettes or humidicribs). Others who are very tiny or seriously ill are on special heated consoles, attached to various tubes and wires, surrounded by monitors, with a nurse for each baby.

Nicola is quite well, although small. She weighs 3.1 kilograms, having been just 2.2 kilograms when she was born three weeks ago. She has been feeding and growing well, doing all the right things. It seems to her mother such a setback for Nicola to have this hernia that needs an operation.

Nicola and her mother settle into the ward. The nurse attaches name tags to Nicola's wrist and ankle and then takes down all the details about her birth and subsequent development, including her feeding pattern and if she has required any medications or had any immunisations.

Very soon, Dr Solomon, the anaesthetist, comes to see them. He asks Nicola's mother the same questions again, as well as asking her about her own experiences with anaesthesia. All appears to be normal. He listens to Nicola's heart and lungs with his stethoscope and checks her weight and temperature chart. The nurse has already applied some local anaesthetic cream to the backs of both Nicola's hands and covered them with a clear plastic dressing.

In response to questions from Dr Solomon as to whether or not she is happy with everything, Nicola's mother becomes a little tearful and asks if Nicola will be all right.

'She's so tiny, isn't it dangerous?'

'There are risks with anaesthesia at all ages,' replies Dr Solomon, taking a chair and sitting down beside her. 'In looking after someone Nicola's age and size, we are careful to measure the doses of all the drugs so that she gets exactly the right amounts, and all the equipment we use is designed especially for someone her size. As you might imagine, we also give anaesthetics to premature babies who are very ill and much smaller than Nicola. That's why you've come to a children's hospital, where we deal with children and babies like Nicola every day.'

'Well, thanks, that does help to reassure me.'

Dr Solomon smiles at her and then adds, 'As part of her anaesthetic I'll be putting in a type of epidural. Did you have one during your labour and delivery with Nicola?'

'Yes,' replies Nicola's mother, 'it worked brilliantly; but is it necessary, or safe, in someone as tiny? I thought she was having a general anaesthetic?'

'She is indeed having a general anaesthetic first, and then once she is asleep, I'll put an injection of long-acting local anaesthetic into the base of her spine. It's a type of epidural, but without the long fine plastic tube that you probably had. We call this a *caudal* anaesthetic. Nicola will have a single injection of local anaesthetic, which will numb the nerves that supply the area of the operation. This will help during the operation, so that she won't need as much general anaesthetic and will recover more quickly. More importantly, the caudal will make sure that Nicola doesn't have any pain for the first four or five hours after the operation.'

'But is it safe?'

'Yes, it is quite safe—it's a very common method of providing excellent pain relief. Most likely Nicola will only need some paracetamol or acetominophen when the local wears off. That means that she probably won't need an injection of a stronger drug like morphine, which is a good pain reliever but which can also decrease the rate of breathing.'

'How long after the operation before she'll be awake?'

'She should be awake within half an hour of the end of the operation—although there is a very small risk with babies who are very tiny or who were born prematurely that they forget to breathe properly after the anaesthetic.'

'What happens then?' asks Nicola's mother, worriedly.

'If that were to happen, then I would stay with Nicola until she is breathing properly and I am absolutely satisfied that it is safe for her to come back to the ward. This is a rare problem in some of these babies, due to their young brains forgetting to breathe. Very rarely we need to leave a little plastic tube in the mouth or nose to help with breathing for them, for a few hours after an anaesthetic. In any case, we like to monitor the breathing of babies like Nicola for at least 12 hours afterwards, just to be sure that everything's okay.'

'Won't she starve? She hasn't had a feed since three this morning.'

'We will be careful not to let her get dehydrated or hungry. I'll be putting in an intravenous line so that we can give her some fluid and sugar if necessary. It's quite likely, though, that she'll be able to be breast-fed before 10 a.m., in other words within an hour of the operation.'

'That will make both of us feel better,' says Nicola's mother. 'Can I be with her until she goes to sleep?'

'I'd prefer not,' answers Dr Solomon. 'At her age, your presence is not so critical. Babies just like to be cuddled and I know she would rather be cuddled by you than by anyone else. Nevertheless, she won't be too upset being separated from you. Children over about the age of six months, on the other hand, do resent being taken away from their mothers. In any case, my job is to look after her. I don't want to have to look after both of you. She deserves my 100 per cent attention, and that's what she's going to get—

until the operation is over and she's safely in the Recovery Room, breathing well on her own.'

RICHARD

Richard makes an appointment and duly attends Dr McKenzie's clinic two weeks later. This time, his daughter, a former nurse, comes with him.

Dr McKenzie ushers Richard and his daughter in, and goes through Richard's history. He then examines his chest, listening with his stethoscope, and measures his blood pressure. He examines Richard's throat and the mobility of his neck and jaw. He also examines his hands. He asks Richard to step on some scales.

'You really are very fit for your age,' says Dr McKenzie. 'It will stand you in good stead. Are you allergic to anything?'

'No,' replies Richard.

'What about medications—you've been on a few anti-inflammatory drugs haven't you?'

'Yes,' says Richard, and reeled off a list of painkillers and anti-inflammatory drugs he had been taking.

'Any trouble with your stomach—with ulcers or heartburn?' asks Dr McKenzie. 'Sometimes those drugs play havoc with your insides.'

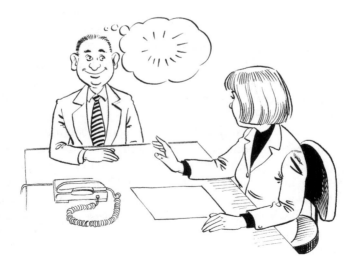

'No, not that I'm aware of.'

'Any other medications?'

'Just a sleeping pill—I started taking them when my wife died and I've been taking them ever since—just two a night.'

'What sort?'

'A little pink one—sorry, that's the one I forgot to bring with me.'

'I didn't know that you took a sleeping pill, Dad,' said his daughter, who until now had sat quietly.

'Almost forgot myself—get into bed, take two, turn off the light, roll over, and go to sleep.'

'Have you ever managed sleeping without them?' asks Dr McKenzie.

'Oh, no. I tried to stop taking them and it was terrible—couldn't sleep a wink and the family wondered why I was so grumpy. Probably should have tried harder to get off them—but it seemed too unpleasant.' His daughter looks at him sympathetically but says nothing.

'Well,' says Dr McKenzie, 'that sometimes causes a bit of a problem after anaesthesia in someone of your age. It's a bit like withdrawal and can occasionally cause a bit of mental confusion.'

'I'm not sure I like the sound of that,' says Richard.

'Nor I,' whispers his daughter.

'We can help with other medication, but it can be a trying time for all, especially your family. Most patients who are a bit confused postoperatively don't remember being so, and it doesn't worry them so much. We'll have to keep an eye on that, if you decide to go ahead with the operation.'

'What about the anaesthetic—isn't it dangerous to put an old chap like me to sleep?'

'In the past it probably was, but now with modern drugs and more information about exactly what we're giving to you, better equipment and techniques, we can very safely look after people like you for major surgery. Clearly, the older you are, the fewer reserves you have and the more likely complications are to occur. Things like heart failure, blood clots in the legs, bronchitis, and pneumonia are more common in older patients. I notice that you wear dentures, so there's no possibility of damaging your teeth.'

Richard takes a deep breath and then says, 'My wife died after an anaesthetic.'

Dr McKenzie responds, 'I'm awfully sorry to hear that. How long ago did she die and what was she having done?'

'She had her gall bladder removed 20 years ago—got pneumonia and never got out of hospital.'

'Well,' comments Dr McKenzie, 'things are certainly a lot better now. We didn't monitor oxygen then, except to observe if the patient was pink. We're also much better at managing patients post-operatively. It's not uncommon for patients after gall bladder surgery to have some difficulty with breathing after the operation, especially if they have to have the big incision, instead of keyhole surgery. The problem is that the incision's right under the lung and every time the patient takes a breath it hurts. So you have an elderly patient, perhaps prone to asthma or bronchitis, who has her breathing and coughing restricted for a few days. Before you know it, pneumonia sets in—and it can be very difficult to diagnose and to treat. But today we're much more aware of how to prevent and, if necessary, how to manage these complications.'

After a pause Richard asks, 'What sort of anaesthetic will you use? I've heard of these operations being done under local.'

'What I would advise is an epidural—the sort of anaesthetic we often use for childbirth.'

Richard's daughter concurs. 'Yes, Dad, you'd be so much better with an epidural.'

'I must say it's easier when someone else is persuading the patient about epidurals. But you need to know a few facts before making up your mind.' Dr McKenzie continues, 'Having an epidural means that we'd put you on your side, wash off your back with some cold antiseptic solution, then inject some freezing into the skin in the middle of your lower back. That feels like a tiny insect bite. Then I'll insert a long needle in between the bones of your spine until I reach the epidural space. That shouldn't hurt at all but you might feel some pressure sensation, which might be a little uncomfortable. You'll need to lie very still while I position the needle carefully and then slide in a fine plastic tube through the needle and into your back. This tube's a bit like fine spaghetti and sometimes it just gently nudges a nerve—it might feel like a small electric shock, or like hitting your funny bone. The important thing is not to move if you feel that, but simply to tell me. Once the catheter's in place, I pull the needle out, and then you can move a little. After I've taped the catheter onto your back, I'll inject a small dose of local anaesthetic to make sure that the catheter hasn't entered a blood vessel. Once I'm sure that everything's okay, then I'll inject more local anaesthetic down through the tube. That might feel like cold liquid running down your back.'

Dr McKenzie continues, 'The beauty of epidural anaesthesia is that we can keep using it for a few days after the operation to keep you really comfortable, without giving you large doses of drugs like morphine. So, above the waist, so to speak, you can be your usual self.'

'What if it doesn't work?'

'I always have the option of giving you a general anaesthetic— which I'm happy to do. But I think that your recovery will be a little quicker with an epidural. In my hands, the epidural works in about 98 per cent of cases, and I won't allow you to suffer any pain during the operation. I will probably give you a small amount of sedation, just so you're not bothered by all the noise and lights, and so on, in the theatre. And if you have a favourite recording and a Walkman, you can wear the earphones and listen to whatever you like. Now, did the surgeon mention you giving some blood ahead of time, so that you don't have to receive anyone else's blood?'

Richard turns to his daughter and asks, 'Was that the appointment at the hospital or at the Red Cross?'

His daughter answers, 'At the Red Cross. The hospital appointment's for you to see the physio.'

'Good,' says Dr McKenzie. 'But you'll still need to have a few tests, if you decide to go ahead. Do you have any questions or concerns, either of you?'

'I think I'm reasonably happy,' replies Richard.

His daughter nods. 'I want him to spend a week or two with us when he gets out of hospital.'

'And who's going to look after my garden?' asks Richard, a little crossly.

'We all will, Dad, we promise. Even the twins will help.'

At the thought of his nine-year-old granddaughters, Richard smiles again.

'Now remember to keep taking all of your medications, especially your blood pressure tablets, and bring them with you to the hospital. We'll get you in the day before. It's too difficult for you to get here for seven o'clock in the morning, and we want to do some tests anyway. About the sleeping tablets, we've got a couple of weeks before the operation. If you can perhaps break the tablets and just take one tablet each night over the next week and then maybe half each night of the following week, it would be helpful for all of us. If you have any questions or concerns over the next couple of weeks, please don't hesitate to give me a call.'

'Thanks, Doctor, I'll remember.'

Two weeks later, Richard is admitted to hospital, just after midday and, as Dr McKenzie had explained, proceeds to have a number of tests. Dr McKenzie arrives to visit in the early evening and checks all the results, looks at the X-ray, and records the information on the chart. He notes that Richard's blood pressure is a little high but not unduly so for an 87-year-old, that his haemoglobin is a little low at 11, and that there was a little sugar in the urine sample. Dr McKenzie decides that he will check Richard's blood sugar during the anaesthetic.

Dr McKenzie asks how Richard has managed with the reduced sleeping pill.

'Not very well—I'm still taking one tablet.'

'Okay, we'll prescribe one for tonight and I'll also make sure you get your blood pressure tablets in the morning.'

SUSAN

Susan's operation is to be performed at ten o'clock, and she is advised to attend the hospital at eight the same morning. She has received a letter from the hospital a week earlier with instructions as to what clothes, etc., she should bring, where to go, and importantly, what she should and should not eat and drink the day before and the day of the operation.

Susan is met by the ward nurse, who escorts her to her room.

Having taken Susan's blood pressure, pulse and temperature, the nurse asks Susan to step onto some scales.

Embarrassed, Susan exclaims, 'I seem to have put on a few pounds since the fibroids were diagnosed—I'm not usually that weight. Does everyone have to go through this?'

'Yes,' says the nurse. 'We need to know your weight because all the drugs and medications are adjusted for your weight. Your anaesthetist in particular will want to know exactly what you weigh.'

'When will I meet the anaesthetist? That's what I'm really worried about.'

'According to the Operating Room schedule, it's Dr Wong this morning, and he always comes around about an hour before surgery. So he should be here soon.'

About ten minutes later, Dr Wong appears and introduces himself to Susan and her husband, Eric.

'Hello, I'm Raymond Wong, your anaesthetist, and I'll be looking after you today while Dr Reitz does the operation. You're having a hysterectomy, is that right?'

'Yes, and I'm more worried about the anaesthetic than the operation,' says Susan.

'Well, it's my job to make sure that you don't need to worry— either of you. I'm there to look after you during the whole time you are in surgery. Have you had any anaesthetics before?'

'No, this is the first time.'

'Have there been any family problems with anaesthetics?'

'Yes, my mother's aunt, my great-aunt, died during an operation—they said she couldn't take the anaesthetic. The family always talk about it whenever there's an operation on TV.'

'Perhaps we can sort out what happened? Do you know much about it—was she old, young, was she sick?'

'The only thing I know is that it was a long time ago, before I was born, and I guess she must have been in her fifties or sixties. Apparently she just didn't wake up afterwards.'

'Do you know what operation she was having?'

'No, I'm not sure—my mother would know but she's away at the moment, visiting my brother out in the country.'

'Has your mother had any anaesthetics?'

'Oh yes, she's had quite a few and they don't seem to worry her. She bounces back and now she's fit as a fiddle.'

'What operations has she had?'

'Let's see—there was the bowel obstruction. I think she'd had her appendix out when she was a little girl. Then she had to have a *colostomy* and then they fixed that up. But she's really good for her age—hope I'm the same when I'm her age.'

'Well, the problem with your great-aunt doesn't sound like anything hereditary then, and certainly the chances of not waking up were much greater with anaesthetics fifty years ago than they are now. I'll keep that information in mind during your anaesthetic and recovery, but unless there's some other specific information, I think we can fairly safely ignore your great-aunt. And you've been perfectly well otherwise—no colds or flu recently?'

'I had a bout of the flu—maybe it was just a bad cold—a couple of weeks ago, but that's all cleared up.'

'Okay. Now are you taking any tablets or medicines?'

'Only the Pill.'

'Right, and which one is it—one of the low-dose ones?'

'I'm not sure. Eric, can you get the packet out of my bag?'

Dr Wong checks the oral contraceptive and determines that it is indeed a low-dose type. He makes another note on the chart on which he has been jotting throughout the interview.

'Now, I'll need to examine you a bit—have a listen to your heart and lungs, and look at your mouth—what we anaesthetists call the airway. And you are right-handed, yes?'

Susan nods in agreement.

Dr Wong first takes Susan's hand, feels her pulse, and then runs an index finger over one of the veins on the back of Susan's left hand.

'Now, to start the anaesthetic, I'll be putting in an intravenous or drip, you know, a little plastic needle into this vein on the back of your hand here.'

'Won't that hurt?' asks Susan worriedly.

'No, because we've got enough time for the nurse to put some local anaesthetic cream on, as soon as I've finished examining you. The cream will make it numb, so you should only notice some slight pressure as I slide the needle in.'

Dr Wong looks at Susan's jaw and asks her to open her mouth, and then to stick out her tongue. He has noticed while speaking with her that she has prominent front teeth and a slightly receding lower jaw. He looks in at the roof of her mouth (*palate*) and observes that it is narrow and that her two front upper teeth slightly overlap each other. He then has her protrude her lower jaw so that her lower teeth rest in front of her upper teeth. After asking Susan to relax her jaw, he places three fingers of his right hand under Susan's jaw.

'What are you doing?' Susan asks.

'I'm measuring the distance from the edge of your lower jaw to the top of the *thyroid cartilage* or Adam's apple here in your neck. What I've been doing is what we anaesthetists call "assessing the airway"—checking how wide your mouth and throat are and determining whether or not we might have any trouble inserting a breathing tube in through your mouth and down into your wind-pipe or trachea. I need to do that as part of the anaesthetic—to take over your breathing and ensure that the passage for oxygen is clear. That won't be done until you're unconscious, so you won't know the tube is going in, and it should be out by the time you're fully conscious again.'

'How do you get the tube in?' asks Eric, who until now has not said anything.

'I'll be using a special instrument called a *laryngoscope*. It's like a big tongue depressor with a special light attached, so that I can see where to place the tube.' Dr Wong turns to Susan and continues. 'The laryngoscope goes into your mouth once you're unconscious and I use it to hold your tongue to the left in your mouth and also to pull your lower jaw forward. Just as I had you do just now, when you moved your lower teeth in front of your upper teeth.'

'Is that what causes the sore throat afterwards? My girlfriend had the same operation about two years ago and she said the worst of it was the sore throat. Does the tube itself do any damage?'

'Well, you've really asked two questions. First, getting the tube in does put some pressure on the tissues inside your throat and I think that's what causes the sore throat. In some patients it's neces-sary to pull the jaw forward more strongly than in others, so there's a bit more pressure on the soft tissues in there. In your case, your lower jaw moves well forward of your upper jaw, and the distance

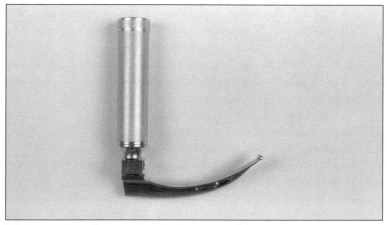

Figure 3   A laryngoscope. The handle contains batteries. The curved 'blade' with the light at the tip is inserted into the mouth as far as the epiglottis, enabling the anaesthetist to see the larynx and insert an endotracheal tube.

I measured under your chin looks just about normal, so I don't think I'll have to pull too hard. As for the tube itself, you might be a little hoarse for a day, but it shouldn't be any worse than that.'

Dr Wong then asks, 'Have you had any special dental work done?'

'I had a chip fixed on one of these front teeth.' She gets out a mirror from her purse and says, 'Yes, the left front one. Otherwise they're all mine, not even a filling!'

'I'll need to watch that,' replies Dr Wong. 'There's always a slight chance of damage to teeth, and veneers or bridges are less strong that most natural teeth, although there's also a risk with brittle or previously chipped teeth. I'll be doing my best to avoid any pressure on your teeth, but I should just let you know. I've drawn a little picture of exactly which tooth has the veneer, so not only will I know, but also the nurses who look after you in the Recovery Room.'

'Thanks! I need these. I do a bit of amateur theatre and people say what a perfect smile I have.'

'I'd like to examine your chest. Would you like your husband to stay or to go out?'

'I'm perfectly happy for him to stay, if it's all right with you.'

'Yes, thank you. Now, if you could just remove your dressing gown so that I can listen to the back of your chest.'

Dr Wong uses his stethoscope to listen to Susan's lungs, and then slips the stethoscope around the front of her chest, listening to her heart.

'Fine, all clear.'

'Do you have the results of my blood tests which I had last week? I think I had something called a cross-match.'

'All your test results are normal. And as for your cross-match, you're A positive.'

'Does that mean I'll be given a blood transfusion?'

'You will lose some blood during the operation, although probably not very much, so it's very unlikely that you will be given blood. Our surgeon likes to have some compatible blood on hand, in case there's heavier bleeding than anticipated. However, I try not to transfuse patients unless they really need it.

'I do need to explain a couple of other things,' Dr Wong goes on. 'Because you are having a hysterectomy, you have an increased risk of a blood clot or *deep vein thrombosis* (DVT) in the legs. This risk is increased because you are on the Pill. We'll be giving you a couple of doses of a drug to thin your blood and also have you wear some fancy stockings. Both of these things should help to prevent any clots. In addition, the sooner you get up and walk about after the operation, the better.'

'I'll certainly try to do that.'

'We also need to plan your recovery, especially as far as pain relief goes. This operation can be very painful afterwards. You're going to have a big cut in your tummy. There are a couple of ways that we can provide pain relief. One is with injections into your bottom. Another is with injections through the intravenous, which you control by pushing a special button whenever you want some more drug. Many patients like this technique, because they get a dose whenever they need it, rather than whenever the nurse is able to get to them. That's why we call it *patient-controlled analgesia* or PCA. And there's very little risk of having too much drug, or an overdose, as the pump has a computer that is programmed to give a specific dose and no more. It's a bit like a bank machine—

you can't take out a thousand dollars every five minutes. Same thing with this pump. The third option for pain relief is with a little tube placed in the middle of your back—an epidural. We can give you small amounts of local anaesthetic and painkiller, such as morphine.'

'Like I had for our first baby. It worked very well, but I was never really happy and I only needed the gas for our second. Though I think might have had an injection as well. I just don't like the idea of having a needle in my back. If I had a choice, then I'd rather have the pump.'

'Fine, then I'll book one for you.'

Eric asks, 'You mean there isn't a pump for every patient?'

'No,' replies Dr Wong. 'In fact, we like to make sure that the patients who really need the pumps get them.'

TOBY

Toby's operation was arranged by the ear, nose, and throat surgeon after Toby spent a night in hospital having his breathing monitored. Part of this sleep study involved measuring the oxygen in Toby's blood, using a special clip like a clothes-peg attached to a thumb, called a pulse oximeter. (This is also part of normal monitoring during anaesthesia.) In Toby's case, the oximetry was carried out to help determine the severity of his obstructive sleep apnoea. This is a condition where people stop breathing while asleep, because of blockage of the upper part of the throat. Each time the person stops breathing, he or she has a period of not getting enough oxygen. Sleep apnoea patients often have noisy and restless sleep as they snore, gag, and splutter, and the brain tells them that they're not getting enough oxygen.

Toby's condition is caused by his enlarged tonsils and adenoids. These are glands in the throat and the back of the nose, which mop up infections. But these glands themselves can become the seat of repeated infections, as in Toby's case. Then they need to be removed.

Toby is overweight. He doesn't sleep very well and is tired during the day, so he doesn't take part in many sports at school. He likes computer games, however, and has brought his handheld game to hospital.

Toby's parents have discussed the operation with him, but he doesn't say much. He's actually quite frightened inside, even afraid of dying or having something dreadful happen to him, like having his insides pulled out while he's asleep. These fears of death or mutilation are not uncommon at his age, but are rarely discussed openly.

Toby has missed his breakfast, too, which doesn't make him happy. He ate some biscuits last night before bed, and he had a drink of apple juice this morning as soon as he got up at half-past six.

Toby and his parents proceed to the surgical admission centre, where the nurse welcomes them and points out the playroom full of toys and video games, as well as a tank brimming with brightly coloured tropical fish.

The first thing the nurse does is weigh Toby. Next she enquires about Toby's medications and whether he has any allergies. Alan says, laughing, that Toby is allergic to spinach.

'What sort of reaction does he have?' asks the nurse.

'Well, none, he just doesn't like it,' replies Alan.

'Oh, that sort of allergy!' responds the nurse, smiling at Toby. 'I meant real allergies—leading to rashes and other reactions.'

After learning that Toby does not have any allergies, the nurse asks other questions about his eating habits, sleep patterns, favourite toys, etc. Then she applies a white cream to the backs of both of his hands and covers the cream with clear, adhesive plastic film.

'This is local anaesthetic cream,' she explains. 'When the anaesthetist uses a small needle, it won't hurt because your skin will be numb.'

Toby is not too sure.

'The anaesthetist, Dr Hansen, will be along to see you shortly.'

Sure enough, Dr Hansen arrives and introduces herself. She explains to Toby what an anaesthetist is: 'The doctor who looks after you during your operation and makes sure that you stay asleep until it's all over.'

She then asks if Toby has had any previous anaesthetics or if there have been any problems in the family with having anaesthetics. She also asks if Toby has had any major illnesses, takes any medications, or has any allergies. Spinach is not mentioned. Dr Hansen asks about the sleep apnoea to find out how severe the breathing problem is, then asks Toby to open his mouth wide and to tip his head back as far as he can. She takes her stethoscope and listens to Toby's chest, front and back. She also takes Toby's hand and explains about the needle and how it won't sting because of the cream. She invites Alan and Jenny to accompany Toby until he falls asleep with the anaesthetic.

Dr Hansen also explains that Toby will have a sore throat after the operation, and that nausea and vomiting are common after operations to remove the tonsils and adenoids. She states that she will administer enough painkillers to make Toby comfortable but not enough to entirely get rid of all his pain as that may lead to a decrease in his rate of breathing. She also indicates that she will give a combination of drugs to try to prevent the nausea and vomiting.

'But I can't guarantee that he won't be sick afterwards. One of the reasons is that there will be a little blood in his stomach—from the tonsils. And it may be enough to make him vomit, possibly just once, to get rid of the blood.'

She then asks if Toby and his parents have any questions, but none are forthcoming. Dr Hansen detects that Toby is quite anxious. She asks if a sedative might help, but Jenny says that Toby will be calm if she can stay with him until he is anaesthetised. Finally Dr Hansen prescribes some mild painkiller (paracetamol or acetaminophen) for Toby to drink before the operation. That done, Dr Hansen leaves and Toby returns to his computer game.

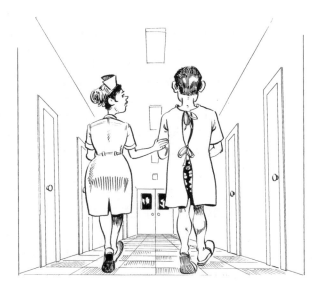

Chapter 7

During your anaesthetic

MEETING YOUR ANAESTHETIST

You may have already met your anaesthetist in the Preoperative Assessment Clinic. If not, then you will meet shortly before you enter the Operating Room. This meeting may take place on a ward, in an admissions unit, or in a holding area outside the Operating Room.

Your anaesthetist has reviewed the information contained in your hospital record or chart, such as the results of any tests you have undergone. He or she asks you some additional questions, such as your or your relatives' experience with anaesthetics. Your anaesthetist talks to you about possible choices of anaesthetic, such as between general and regional or local anaesthesia, and about any specific problems or concerns you have. In addition, your anaesthetist discusses with you the different choices for post-operative pain management.

After this, your anaesthetist examines you, by looking at your mouth, your teeth, and the veins of your hands, arms, and neck, and may listen to your chest. If you are to have a regional or local anaesthetic, your anaesthetist also looks at the area of your body where the anaesthetic is to be injected, such as the small of your back.

This is your opportunity to ask about your anaesthetic. Even though you may think that the time for questions is short, you should ask whatever you want and make sure that all your questions are answered.

WHERE DO I 'GO TO SLEEP'?

In some hospitals, you are taken directly into the Operating Room and then given your anaesthetic. In other hospitals, you are taken into a smaller room adjacent to the Operating Room. This smaller room is known as the Anaesthetic Induction Room, as it is where the anaesthetic is 'induced' or started.

A few general statements can be made. First, when you enter the Operating Room or Anaesthetic Induction Room, you have what are termed 'routine monitors' attached. These monitors are used for virtually every patient and include an ECG (electrocardiograph), a pulse oximeter probe, and a blood pressure cuff. In addition, in most cases an intravenous line is started, usually in a vein in the back of one of your hands or in a vein in your forearm.

Second, there are three phases to any anaesthetic:

- **Start or induction phase:** The anaesthetist gives you the drugs that make you lose consciousness, in the case of a general anaesthetic; or performs the *nerve block* that makes part of you numb (as in a spinal or an epidural).
- **Middle or maintenance phase:** The anaesthetist ensures that you remain anaesthetised until the surgical, diagnostic, or treatment procedure is completed.
- **End or emergence phase:** The anaesthetist stops giving you the anaesthetic drugs, allows them to wear off, and/or gives you other drugs to reverse their effects, so that you regain consciousness or sensation.

KEEPING A RECORD

While monitoring your anaesthetic, your anaesthetist keeps a record of your vital signs, such as your heart rate, blood pressure, and oxygen saturation. Your anaesthetist also records the time, dose, and route of all drugs and fluids that you are given. A record may also be made of routine and special monitors and equipment, as well as any anaesthetic techniques. As well, your anaesthetist makes a note of any events of importance. These might include, for example, the time when your surgeon made the first incision or other important actions.

Exactly what your anaesthetist records partly reflects local custom. For example, in Canada the *Guidelines to the Practice of Anaesthesia* describe the minimum amount of information that should be recorded. Similar guidelines exist in Australia, New Zealand, and other countries. These guidelines state that every patient undergoing general, regional, or monitored anaesthesia care should have his or her blood pressure and heart rate measured and recorded at least every five minutes. There is one important exception to this statement, which is contained in the phrase 'unless clinically impractical'. This phrase applies if your condition is very unstable and your anaesthetist is working hard to save your life—for example, giving you life-saving drugs and intravenous fluids. In this case, your anaesthetist might not be able to record your blood pressure or heart rate at the same time. If so, your anaesthetist would complete the anaesthetic record after the crisis was over and your condition had stabilised.

GENERAL ANAESTHESIA

'Going off to sleep' (induction phase)

As described earlier, the first phase of an anaesthetic is known as the induction phase. Your anaesthetist may start your anaesthetic or induce 'sleep' in one of three ways. Induction may be:

- intravenous (into the vein): the most common method
- inhalation (by breathing in): often used in children
- intramuscular (into the muscle) injection: now used very rarely.

Intravenous induction

Before having an intravenous induction, you may have had local anaesthetic cream applied to the skin over the vein to be used for the initial injection. The location of the vein depends on the anaesthetist's preference, the site of the operation, and the appearance of your veins. Often the veins on the back of the hand or forearm are used. The choice of hand depends on whether you are left- or right-handed, because having a bruise on the back of your dominant hand may cause discomfort afterwards. Also, if your intravenous line must remain in place for some time, you will find it easier to be able to do things, such as combing your hair or brushing your teeth, if your intravenous is not in the hand with which you normally do these things.

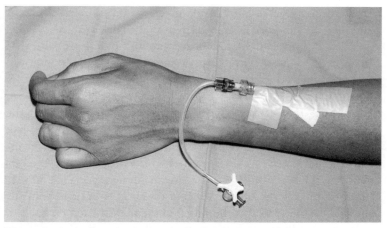

Figure 4   An intravenous cannula. During insertion of the cannula, the outer plastic tube is closely fitted to an inner hollow needle. Having inserted the tip of the needle into the vein, the plastic cannula is pushed off the needle and into the vein. The needle is then removed and discarded. Plastic tubing and injection taps may then be attached for administration of drugs or fluids.

Having wiped away the cream and applied some alcohol to the skin, your anaesthetist inserts a cannula or fine plastic tube into the vein. This is accompanied by a sensation varying between slight pain and a feeling of light pressure. In the absence of local anaesthetic cream, you feel a short sharp pain. The cannula is secured to the skin with tape and may be attached to an intravenous 'line' or long clear plastic tube connected to a bag of saline or similar fluid. This fluid may feel cold when it runs into the vein (usually in your arm).

Your anaesthetist may then have you breathe oxygen from a mask. This process is known as preoxygenation. This mask is attached by tubing to the anaesthetic machine. Because the tubing or mask may be a type of rubber, it may give off a chemical smell. This smell is from the anaesthetic gases which have diffused into the rubber.

Your anaesthetist may also give you one or more drugs, before giving you the actual drug which makes you lose consciousness. For example, if you are booked to have your gall bladder removed, your anaesthetist might start by giving you an injection of a drug to relax you, and then a drug to decrease the chance of postoperative vomiting. You might also be given an injection of a potent painkiller (or narcotic), such as fentanyl. This drug also helps minimise any marked rises in heart rate and blood pressure that can occur at a slightly later stage of the anaesthetic and operation. Sometimes anaesthetists give these additional drugs after you have lost consciousness.

The anaesthetist then injects the induction drug through the cannula into your vein. This is the time when he or she may ask you to count (often backwards, from 100). Counting is a means of distracting you and also shows when the drug has achieved its effect. It works very quickly, especially in younger patients. It takes only the time for the blood carrying the drug to return from the arm to the heart and then be pumped through the lungs, back to the heart, and then to the brain. (Anaesthetists call this the 'arm–brain circulation time'.) In most people this time is about ten seconds, but it may be faster in children and slower in elderly or very ill patients.

How does my anaesthetist know how much to give me?

Individuals vary in their requirements for anaesthetic drugs. The dose of the induction drug is generally given slowly to patients who are to have an elective operation. Your anaesthetist has calculated the expected dose you should need, from your weight, your age, your sex, and your state of health. However, as the drugs are injected, the dose of each is adjusted as necessary, according to the effects produced. This is known as *titrating* the drugs according to their effect. In an emergency it is sometimes necessary to give the drugs quickly, and a predetermined dose is calculated.

Will I have the same anaesthetic as the patient in the bed next to me?

Every anaesthetic given is a very individual thing and each anaesthetic depends on the patient to whom it is given. The doses of drugs that you are given are calculated according to your weight, age, and state of health; the operation or examination for which they are given; and the anaesthetist who gives them. In a department or practice of ten anaesthetists, there may be ten different approaches to general anaesthesia. There is no fixed recipe.

Inhalation (gas) induction

This method is common in children but is also used in some adults. It involves having the anaesthetist or the patient hold a mask over the patient's nose and mouth. The patient then breathes in a mixture of gases through the face mask until loss of consciousness occurs. Induction by mask usually takes longer than the intravenous method, and achievement of the appropriate depth of anaesthesia is often preceded by a period of restlessness. This is quite normal and the patient is already unconscious at this time.

Then the anaesthetist has an assistant (nurse, technician, or another anaesthetist) hold the mask and ensure that the patient is continuing to breathe well. The anaesthetist then inserts an intravenous cannula (as above), unless one has previously been started. This is more likely to have been done in adults. From this point, the anaesthetic is similar, whether an intravenous or inhalation technique has been used.

Establishing an airway

After the induction drug has caused you to lose consciousness, your anaesthetist gives you one or more other drugs (a mixture of narcotics and anaesthetic gases) to ensure that you remain unconscious. If these other anaesthetic agents were not given, you would regain

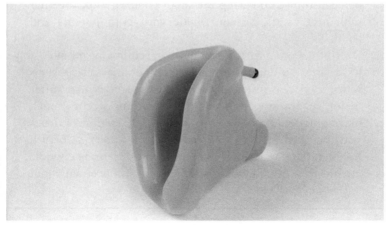

Figure 5   A face mask. The inflatable cushion provides comfort as well as an airtight seal around the mouth and nose.

consciousness in a few minutes, after the induction drug had worn off.

Your anaesthetist then takes over the management of your breathing, while attending to any changes in your pulse, blood pressure, and the amount of oxygen in the blood. This management might consist of holding the mask over your mouth and nose, ensuring that you are breathing clearly and without snoring; or holding the mask and breathing for you by squeezing a bag attached to the breathing circuit; or inserting a breathing tube into your mouth.

INDUCTION OF ANAESTHESIA IN CHILDREN

Children vary greatly in the way they react to induction of anaesthesia. All children exhibit fear in some way, because of the strange environment, separation from their parents, and the uncertainty about what is to happen to them.

LESS THAN SIX MONTHS

Infants of less than six months do not react strongly to being separated from their parents and usually respond appropriately to a parent substitute. The anaesthetist should be accustomed to caring for small children and, together with other staff, be empathetic with both parents and child.

It is uncommon for parents to accompany infants of less than six months during induction of anaesthesia. This is for two reasons: a child of this age does not suffer major separation anxiety; and everything occurs much more quickly in a baby. This includes the action of drugs and the need to act to correct problems such as breath holding. The anaesthetist must devote his or her whole attention to the child without having to be concerned about parents as well.

SIX MONTHS TO FOUR YEARS

Children in this age group do not tolerate separation from their parents well and are not able to comprehend explanation. They react to the unknown with fear, withdrawal, and struggling. Induction of anaesthesia is best performed either with a parent present, or premedication, or both. With a parent present, the child tends to cling. Induction of anaesthesia can be difficult in this age group. Adequately sedated, there is little problem and usually no recollection of events. However, the sedative drugs may prolong the recovery phase and delay discharge from hospitals after minor or day-stay operations.

With a parent present, either an intravenous or inhalation (gas) induction may be used. For intravenous induction, the parent is asked to hold the child firmly, with the parent either sitting on a chair or leaning over the child who is in a cot or a bed. The parent is then asked to interact with the child by talking, singing, or playing with a toy. At the same time, an assistant secures an arm or a leg where local anaesthetic cream has been applied, while the anaesthetist inserts a cannula.

Inhalation induction is preferred by some anaesthetists. However, usually a mask cannot be placed over a child's face without a struggle. Sometimes this struggle may be minimised by the anaesthetist applying a few drops of a common food flavouring, such as strawberry, orange, or bubblegum, to the mask. These scents help to disguise the smell of the anaesthetic gases. Alternatively, some anaesthetists use their hand as a mask. Induction by mask takes longer than intravenous induction.

FOUR TO SIX YEARS

Children in this age group are still anxious about separation but are more accepting of explanations and reassurance. As with younger children, they benefit from having a parent present during induction, although less physical restraint is required.

SIX TO TEN YEARS

Children aged six to ten years have less of a problem with separation from parents and are much more amenable to reassurance. They do, however, fear anaesthesia and surgery, and particularly pain. They may have fantasies of mutilation and require reassurance about the exact nature of the operation. They may be irritable and impatient.

Intravenous induction is usually well tolerated, although the fear of needles may be so strong that even application of local anaesthetic cream is not enough to overcome the fear. Cooperation can usually be obtained for an inhalation induction with a mask. Sometimes a child indicates a preference, especially if he or she has had previous anaesthetics.

ADOLESCENTS

This group of patients may fear loss of control and death. It is important to reassure them about the safety of modern anaesthesia and that they can be in control of their pain management after the operation.

Intravenous induction is commonly used in adolescents. However, some patients request an inhalation induction, particularly if they have undergone several (or multiple) operations.

YOUR ROLE AS A PARENT DURING INDUCTION OF ANAESTHESIA

You can be an enormous help during induction of your child's anaesthetic. Your presence, in most cases, means a calmer, more cooperative patient, with less likelihood of bad memories of the hospitalisation.

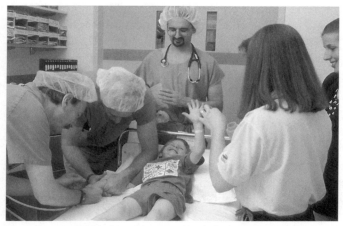

Figure 6   A child having his anaesthetic induced by intravenous injection. His mother is present, and he is distracted by the nurse blowing bubbles. The presence of local anaesthetic cream on the site of injection usually makes the process painless.

There are several points to consider. Just as your child needs to be prepared for the event, so you need to learn as much as you can about what will happen.

Part of your preparation includes recognising that you, too, may be distressed by the experience. The final decision rests with the anaesthetist as to your presence. Although many anaesthetists are used to having parents present at induction, some find their presence stressful. For the child's safety, an anaesthetist may prefer not to have this added distraction.

Your presence may not be encouraged in every situation. This applies particularly if your child needs an emergency operation. Should something happen, such as your child vomiting, then the anaesthetist needs to focus attention on the child.

You should not feel pressured to be involved. Not everyone is comfortable with the idea of staying during induction and you are free to decline the invitation. Your child's care will be no less professional.

You should be prepared for your child's appearance after induction. Your child will become anaesthetised within seconds and may suddenly look lifeless, but often with the eyes still open. This is normal. At the same time the anaesthetist is concentrating on the next step in the process of caring for your child. He or she usually cannot talk with you or answer questions at that time.

You should go when asked to leave.

To help manage your breathing, your anaesthetist might inject a muscle relaxant, to relax or weaken your throat and abdominal muscles. Muscle relaxants have two major useful effects.

- They make it easier for your anaesthetist to insert a breathing (endotracheal) tube through your mouth or, on occasion, through your nose, into your trachea or windpipe. (This process is known as tracheal *intubation*.) Without muscle relaxants, your anaesthetist would have to give higher doses of other drugs so as to weaken the muscles of your mouth and throat, to make insertion of the tube (intubation) easier.
- They actually make it possible for the surgeon to perform many operations, without causing any damage to muscle fibres. Indeed, it is difficult for a surgeon to operate inside your abdomen if the muscles are not relaxed. The same applies to other operations, such as those on the hip or in the chest, but not for those on the skin or the body surface.

If you have been given a muscle relaxant, all of your muscles have been relaxed or weakened, including the muscles that help with breathing. In that case, your anaesthetist 'breathes for you'. This is usually done with a ventilator, which pushes gas around the anaesthetic circuit and into your lungs. Ventilation may also be done by hand, with your anaesthetist squeezing a bag attached to the anaesthetic circuit.

Thus, throughout the operation you are given oxygen, first with a mask over your face, and then through a plastic airway. There are several types of airway, each of which is a different size, depending on your age and size. The presence of an airway helps to ensure that your breathing is adequate and, in the case of an endotracheal (breathing) tube, that acid from your stomach does not pass into your lungs.

The smallest airway is the *oral* airway. An average adult airway is about ten centimetres in length and one centimetre in

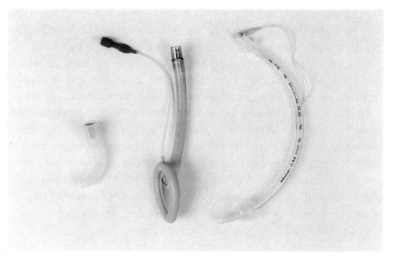

Figure 7 Airways. From left: oral airway, laryngeal mask airway, and endotracheal tube with tracheal cuff inflated.

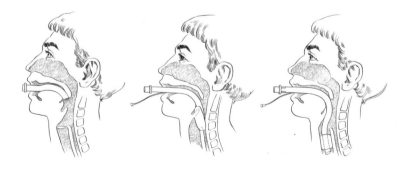

Figure 8 Airways in place. From left: oral airway, laryngeal mask airway, and endotracheal tube.

diameter, and it is curved to fit over the back of the tongue. An oral airway is most often used for minor operations, such as those on a limb, particularly if the duration of the procedure is to be short. The laryngeal mask airway is longer and fits over the top of the larynx. Many anaesthetists now use the laryngeal mask for cases that would previously have had an oral airway and for cases that may have required an endotracheal tube.

The endotracheal tube is long enough to reach from just outside your mouth or nose down to just below your vocal cords. The decision to use an endotracheal tube is determined by your condition, the operation to be performed, and the position in which you are placed during the operation. Your anaesthetist may choose to place a tube if you are very fat, or have a condition known as a hiatus hernia. Usually, an endotracheal tube is used if the surgeon is to operate on the brain, the head and neck region, the chest, the back, the abdomen, or the pelvis. Although the anaesthetic is started while you are lying on your back, your surgeon may need you to be in a different position for the operation. For example, if you are to have an operation on your back, the Operating Room team turn you over onto your stomach after you are unconscious and an endotracheal tube has been inserted.

An airway is placed in your mouth after you become unconscious, although rarely an endotracheal tube must be inserted before any drugs are given and you are still conscious. This is known as 'awake intubation' and is likely if you have a tumour or severe infection in your throat, where the swelling or obstruction makes placement of the tube too risky after you have lost consciousness. In that case, you are given a solution of local anaesthesia to gargle, which numbs your mouth and throat, and decreases any gagging or coughing as the tube is inserted. Some anaesthetists also inject some local anaesthetic through the skin of the neck into your windpipe (trachea), to stop you coughing as the tube is inserted. This is known as a transtracheal injection.

If your anaesthetist has decided that only an oral airway is necessary, then he or she continues to hold the mask over your nose and mouth and connects the mask to the system of hoses called the anaesthetic breathing system or circuit. (Some patients do not have an oral airway inserted and simply breathe from the mask.)

If your anaesthetist has chosen to use a laryngeal mask or an endotracheal tube, it is connected to the circuit after it has been inserted. Your anaesthetist controls and monitors the flow and concentration of gases that enter and leave the circuit and your body, so that you receive the appropriate amount of anaesthetic and breathe adequately.

How does the anaesthetist know that the tube is where it should be?

If the anaesthetist has inserted an endotracheal tube into your trachea (windpipe), you breathe out carbon dioxide through it. (This gas is produced by the body as it uses oxygen to produce

---

MODIFICATION OF THE NORMAL PROCESS OF INDUCTION OF GENERAL ANAESTHESIA

Your anaesthetist might modify the induction of anaesthesia by using a technique known as a *rapid sequence induction* combined with *cricoid pressure*. This is a crucial technique in patients who must undergo an emergency operation and who have a full stomach, either because they have just eaten or because their stomachs take longer than normal to empty (as a result of pain, drugs, or other conditions).

In a rapid sequence induction, you are given 100 per cent oxygen to breathe from a mask placed firmly over your mouth and nose for three to four minutes. This process is known as preoxygenation and replaces the nitrogen in your lungs (the most common gas in the air) with oxygen. As a result, the store of oxygen in your body is markedly increased and there is less chance of lack of oxygen (*hypoxia*).

In the next step your anaesthetist calculates the dose of two drugs—the induction drug (Pentothal or propofol) and a short-acting muscle relaxant, known as suxamethonium (or succinylcholine). The dose of each drug is calculated on the basis of your weight and your general condition.

Your anaesthetist then injects the two drugs rapidly through the intravenous cannula and you quickly lose consciousness. This minimises any risk of your going through a stage during the loss of consciousness when you struggle or vomit.

As you lose consciousness, your anaesthetist instructs an assistant to apply firm pressure to the front of your neck. The assistant normally stands on your right and uses the first three fingers of the right hand to apply the pressure. (You might feel the assistant's fingers lightly touching your neck as you lose consciousness.) The specific part where the pressure is applied, called your cricoid cartilage, is a ring of cartilage that forms part of your trachea. Pressure on the cricoid cartilage (cricoid pressure) seals off the oesophagus and reduces the possibility of stomach contents flowing from the oesophagus into the back of the throat and then down into the lungs.

energy. Carbon dioxide is then excreted from the body through the lungs.) The presence of carbon dioxide suggests that the tube is in your trachea.

There are other methods to help confirm the correct position of the tube, but they are less accurate than the carbon dioxide monitor. Your anaesthetist may also use a stethoscope to listen for the sounds of air moving in and out of your lungs on both sides of your chest, and carefully observe how your chest moves up and down with each breath, noting whether this movement is symmetrical, which usually occurs when the tube is in the trachea.

Your anaesthetist may also listen to your chest to ensure that the tracheal tube has not been placed too far down into one lung. This is known as an *endobronchial intubation* and is sometimes done on purpose. If the surgeon wants to operate on the left lung, the tube is intentionally placed into the right lung.

Maintenance phase

During the maintenance phase of the anaesthetic, your anaesthetist keeps you in a state of unconsciousness, using a mixture of inhaled (inhalational) and intravenous (injected) drugs. The inhalational agents are administered through the breathing circuit. They include nitrous oxide and the 'volatile' anaesthetic agents (because they pass easily from being a liquid to a gas). The volatile anaesthetic agents are commonly used in proportions between 0.5 and 4 per cent, although this varies according to the agent and the desired effect. They are powerful drugs and are used to keep you unconscious, as well as helping to control pain and to relax muscles. These drugs can also have side-effects such as low blood pressure, changes in heart rhythm, and difficulties with breathing.

Nitrous oxide (N_2O) ('laughing gas') is commonly used in most general anaesthetics, in a mixture with oxygen of around 70 per cent nitrous oxide and 30 per cent oxygen. At that concentration the nitrous oxide may make you sleepy and able to tolerate mildly painful procedures, but that is all. Nitrous oxide does, however, provide a means of giving other stronger anaesthetic gases through the breathing system.

Air is sometimes used when nitrous oxide is less desirable, such as during anaesthesia for some brain surgery, for some major heart and lung surgery, and in some tiny premature infants. The medical air is pure and contains the same proportion of oxygen as the air we breathe every day—21 per cent.

During most anaesthetics, however, oxygen is added so that the usual proportion given to the patient is about 30 per cent. This extra oxygen provides some safety margin over the normal 21 per cent in room air. Obviously, the critical aspect of anaesthetic care is to ensure that you continue to receive adequate oxygen, which is necessary for preservation of life and the functioning of organs.

Your anaesthetist may choose to give you other drugs through the intravenous line. Depending on the drug, your anaesthetist may do this to increase the depth of the anaesthetic (how unconscious you are). Narcotics are also given to provide pain relief after the operation. If the surgeon needs your muscles to be relaxed (in order to perform the procedure), your anaesthetist may give you further doses of the muscle relaxant drug given at the time of induction, or a different drug. Intravenously administered drugs may be given in separate or discrete doses (sometimes known as 'bolus' doses) or by constant injection or 'infusion' regulated by a pump.

What else do the anaesthetic drugs do?

Few anaesthetic drugs have single effects. Most cause other changes in the functioning of different parts of the body. For instance, one of the drugs used in general anaesthesia is isoflurane. This drug is administered in a gas mixture and is breathed by the patient. Its intended effect is to maintain the state of unconsciousness and, to a lesser extent, to provide some pain relief. Your anaesthetist administers a higher concentration of the drug to deepen the state of unconsciousness and give more pain relief. As more drug is used, there are other changes in body function that are not primarily intended. These changes include a fall in blood pressure, which may be greater in an elderly patient, in a patient who is dehydrated, or in a patient who has lost blood.

Emergence phase

The third phase of the general anaesthetic is *emergence* or regaining consciousness. During this phase your anaesthetist stops giving you all inhalational anaesthetic agents (except the oxygen) and also stops any intravenous anaesthetic drugs. You gradually regain consciousness. Your anaesthetist usually needs to reverse the effects of the muscle relaxants, with the injection of two more drugs. Measurement of the effectiveness of the muscle relaxant and the degree of reversal is usually performed with a 'nerve stimulator', which is part of the normal anaesthetic monitoring equipment.

As consciousness returns, your anaesthetist makes sure that you can breathe without help. Once you are conscious and able to breathe without any help from the anaesthetist, the breathing tube is removed. By carefully calculating the right amounts of each drug, your anaesthetist can ensure that you are completely unconscious during the operation, but awake and pain-free at the end of the procedure.

REGIONAL ANAESTHESIA

There are many different types of regional anaesthetics. The term regional refers to the fact that only part of the body is anaesthetised. The term *nerve block* means that the transmission of impulses in the nerve or nerves from the area of the operation is blocked by the injection of local anaesthetic agents around the nerve(s). You feel numb or 'frozen' in the area of the block. Local anaesthetics can be administered around the nerves in the spinal cord, either as a spinal or as an epidural anaesthetic. Local anaesthetics can also be injected close to other nerves, such as those in the arms or legs. Because these nerves tend to be in the body's extremities, these nerve blocks may be called peripheral nerve blocks.

Not only are there different types of regional blocks, but there are also different types of local anaesthetics that act for different lengths of time. By choosing various drugs, your anaesthetist can tailor the length of your anaesthetic to match the length of the operation. Sometimes the anaesthetist inserts a fine plastic tube through the nerve block needle. This allows your anaesthetist to give you one or more injections of local anaesthetic, without having to reinsert the needle. This is known as giving a 'top-up'.

Your anaesthetist then checks to see how well the block has worked, by touching your skin with an ice cube or an alcohol swab. If the block has worked, you cannot feel 'cold' when touched. Some anaesthetists use a very fine sterile needle and ask you if the needle feels 'sharp' (where the area supplied by the nerve is not blocked) or 'blunt' (where the nerve is blocked).

The aim of any nerve block is to stop you feeling any pain. However, it is important to remember that you might feel touch, pressure, or vibration, and this is considered normal for certain blocks using certain drugs.

Most anaesthetists like to remind their patients that they may feel 'something' but are very unlikely to feel pain. If the block does not work, there are several options:

- The block can be repeated.
- If the area of sensation is small, the surgeon might be able to inject a small amount of local anaesthetic into the area where you felt the pain.

- Your anaesthetist can give you some medication for pain, such as a low concentration of nitrous oxide or a small amount of an injected narcotic.
- A general anaesthetic may be given instead.
- Finally, in some patients it is better to cancel the procedure and try again another day.

After determining that your block has worked, your anaesthetist helps the nurse to set up the sterile drapes or sheets that separate you from where the surgeon is working. These drapes also prevent you from seeing what is being done. Your anaesthetist continues to monitor how you feel in general, and your vital signs (blood pressure, heart rate, and oxygen saturation). During the course of the procedure, depending on how you are feeling, your anaesthetist might choose to give you an intravenous injection of a sedative, to relax you. You will feel drowsy and might even drift off into what seems like a light sleep. At the end of the operation you will probably not remember much about the events in the Operating Room. When you are transferred to the Recovery Room, you feel relaxed, free of pain, and quite awake.

The choice of which particular block to use is based in part on the anaesthetist's experience and the potential for the block to cause side-effects. The major problems that occur with nerve blocks are related to the needle and to the agent injected. The needle can cause damage to nerves and to other neighbouring structures. For example, a block of the major group of nerves to the arm, when performed at a site just above the collarbone ('supraclavicular approach to the brachial plexus') is associated with a 1 or 2 per cent risk of damage to the lung (pneumothorax). This is because the nerves are close to the outer lining of the lung.

Injection of local anaesthetic agents can cause side-effects because of allergic reactions (see chapter 11) or because of mis-placement of the needle. Because an artery and vein surround each nerve, it is possible to inject local anaesthetic into either of these blood vessels. This results in a sudden increase in the concentration of local anaesthetic in the bloodstream, which can cause convulsions and cardiac arrest. To reduce the chances of these complications, nerve blocks should be performed in the Operating Room or in a specially equipped room where monitors and

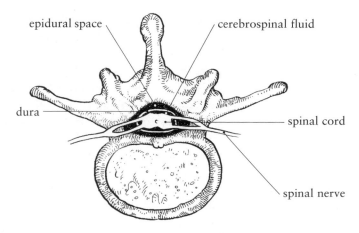

Figure 9   Cross-section of the spinal column, showing layers and structures. For spinal anaesthesia, the drug is placed in the cerebrospinal fluid directly surrounding the spinal cord. For epidural anaesthesia, the drug is placed outside the dura, acting on the spinal nerves as they cross the epidural space.

resuscitation equipment are available. This equipment includes oxygen, a means of delivering the oxygen to the lungs, suction apparatus (in case of vomiting), and items for tracheal intubation. It is vital to have properly trained assistance available.

Spinal and epidural anaesthesia

The most common types of nerve blocks are spinals and epidurals. On their own, either can be used to provide anaesthesia for surgery on the body from about the waist down. The spinal cord is surrounded by fluid within a tough fibrous envelope called the 'dura' (see figure 9). With a spinal, the drug is injected into the fluid. With an epidural, the drug is placed outside the dura, but still within the hollow spinal canal of the backbone.

Spinal anaesthesia

Spinal anaesthetics are useful for surgical procedures involving the legs and lower abdomen. Typical surgical procedures include Caesarean section, vaginal hysterectomy, operations on the prostate, repair of inguinal or groin hernias, repair of a fractured hip, and arthroscopic examination of the knee.

There are a few reasons why you might not be suitable for a spinal anaesthetic. It might be your choice not to have a spinal. The other major reasons have to do with an increased risk of complications from this technique. These include an infection at the site where the needle is inserted, increased pressure around the brain (from a tumour, a build-up of spinal fluid, or the presence of a blood clot) and problems with poor blood clotting. All of these are extremely rare.

If you have a spinal anaesthetic, your anaesthetist first attaches various monitors (ECG, blood pressure cuff, pulse oximeter), and starts an intravenous line. You are then positioned, either lying on one side or sitting up on the edge of the Operating Room table or trolley. If you are lying down, you are asked to curl up into a ball, with your knees drawn up to your chin (or as high as possible). If you are sitting up, you lean over a pillow placed on a small table. In either case, a nurse or the anaesthetist's assistant helps you to get into position and to remain as still as possible. You have a sheet or blanket to cover your chest and the lower half of your body.

Then your anaesthetist feels the bones of your back to choose the level to insert the spinal needle. The site most often chosen is about 4–5 centimetres below your waist and right in the middle ('midline'). After this, your anaesthetist scrubs up, and puts on sterile gloves and perhaps a sterile gown as well. After washing a small area in the middle of your back, using antiseptic solution (which is usually cold), the anaesthetist covers the surrounding skin with sterile cloths.

The next step is insertion of the needle, during which it is extremely important for you to hold as still as possible. Your anaesthetist first gives you a small injection of some local anaesthetic into the area where the spinal needle will be inserted. This injection might feel like a small bee-sting. Then the specially designed spinal needle is inserted into the epidural space and through the covering over the spinal cord (dura). Sometimes there is a tiny 'pop' or 'click' when this happens. Once the spinal needle penetrates the dura, it sits in the spinal canal. This is a sack-like structure containing the cerebrospinal fluid, nerve roots, and the spinal cord. Local anaesthetics (and sometimes a narcotic) are injected into the spinal fluid through the needle, which is then removed.

After the needle is removed, it is safe for you to move a little bit. If you are sitting up, your anaesthetist has you lie down after about 30 seconds. If you are lying down, you continue to lie in that position, although you can straighten your legs and your neck. The local anaesthetic solution disperses in the spinal fluid and blocks the nerves. Over the next few minutes you develop profound numbness and weakness in the lower half of your body (or one side more than the other if the spinal was inserted when you were lying on one side).

The major immediate risks of spinal anaesthetics include nerve damage from the needle, a decrease in blood pressure and heart rate, and failure of the injection to produce an adequate level of anaesthesia. The chance of the block not working is about 1 per cent or less, depending on how frequently your anaesthetist performs spinal blocks.

The long-term complications of spinal anaesthesia include a 1 per cent chance of a severe headache afterwards. Termed a post-dural puncture headache, it is unusual in that it comes on when a patient sits or stands up and is completely resolved by lying down. (The medical term for this phenomenon is 'posturally dependent headache'.) Specific treatment may be needed for the headache. One extremely rare complication includes compression of the spinal cord from a blood clot or abscess in the spinal canal. Another rare complication is ongoing nerve damage from chemical effects of the anaesthetic or other agents on the nerve roots.

A slightly more common complaint is irritation of a nerve root (radicular irritation syndrome). With this problem, patients report burning pain in the legs. The pain comes on a few days after having a spinal with certain local anaesthetic drugs. Fortunately, the pain goes away without any treatment.

Epidural anaesthesia

Like spinal anaesthesia, epidural anaesthesia can be used for operations on the legs and the lower part of the abdomen. Epidurals can also be inserted to help with pain management, either after an operation or during labour.

The technique of insertion of the epidural needle is similar to that used for spinal anaesthesia. However, the needle is stopped in the epidural space and there is no attempt to penetrate the dura. Usually, epidural anaesthesia is performed using a larger needle through which a fine plastic tube (catheter) can be threaded into the epidural space. This tube is similar to fine cooked spaghetti and it is not always possible to determine where the tip of the catheter ends up. Occasionally a patient complains of a brief, shock-like sensation as the catheter is being threaded through the needle and into the back. Most anaesthetists warn their patients that this might happen and remind them not to move until the needle is withdrawn. Once the catheter is well situated, the needle is removed. The catheter is then taped up the back and secured to the hospital gown. A filter is attached to the catheter—in case the fluid to be injected contains tiny particles of glass from the drug ampoules, and to keep bacteria out.

Epidurals are often inserted to relieve the pain of labour and childbirth, as well as postoperative pain. In such cases, epidural analgesia is provided instead of epidural anaesthesia. The only difference between anaesthesia and analgesia is that analgesia uses weaker concentrations of local anaesthetic. A narcotic may also be injected into the epidural to increase pain relief. Epidurals differ from spinals in that a much larger dose of local anaesthetic is required for an epidural anaesthetic as compared to a spinal anaesthetic.

Epidurals can be inserted into the upper part of the back (the thoracic spine), and are then known as thoracic epidurals. These are particularly useful for the relief of postoperative pain after operations on the chest (thoracic surgery). In addition, the anaesthetist may use the pain relief from the epidural to reduce the amount of general anaesthetic needed during the operation.

The immediate risks from epidural anaesthesia include a decrease in blood pressure, and seizures from the accidental intravenous injection of local anaesthetic agents. In addition, effects similar to spinal anaesthesia can be seen, but because of the larger dose of local anaesthetic used with epidurals, the patient may be anaesthetised from the neck down.

The long-term complications of epidural anaesthesia include a less than 1 per cent chance of the block failing to work, and a similar chance of having a post-dural puncture headache. Also possible is damage to a nerve root from the epidural needle or catheter. In extremely rare cases, an epidural blood clot (haematoma) or abscess may occur, resulting in weakness of the legs and in loss of bowel and bladder control.

Other nerve blocks

Other parts or regions of the body can also be anaesthetised ('frozen')—for example, for operations on an eye, arm, or foot. Many different techniques have been described for such operations.

Operations on the eye can be performed under retrobulbar or peribulbar block. These blocks involve injecting local anaesthetic around the eyeball, so that the eye is pain-free and unable to move. This kind of block is used for many operations on the eye, including cataract extraction with lens insertion and repair of defects on the retina (back of the eye). Some cataract operations can also be performed under local anaesthesia, after local anaesthetic drops have been applied to the surface of the eye.

For surgery on the arm it is possible to provide satisfactory anaesthesia by blocking the major group of nerves (brachial nerve plexus) that supplies the shoulder and arm. A block may be performed at one of a number of different sites, including:

- in the neck (interscalene)
- above the collarbone (supraclavicular)
- below the collar bone (infraclavicular)
- in the armpit (axillary).

For surgery on the leg it is possible to provide satisfactory anaesthesia by blocking the major group of nerves (sciatic nerve or femoral nerve) that supplies the hip, leg and foot. A block may be performed at one of several sites, including:

- in the groin (inguinal)
- under the buttocks
- at the back of the knee (popliteal fossa)
- at the ankle.

The intravenous technique, or Bier's block, can be used for operations on the arm, such as reduction of simple fractures of the wrist, and less commonly for procedures on the leg. With this technique, a special tourniquet with two cuffs is wrapped around the arm or leg to be anaesthetised. An intravenous cannula is inserted into a vein in the hand or foot, but no intravenous line is attached. The anaesthetist then lifts up the arm or leg and wraps a tight rubber bandage around it, to drain the blood. The tourniquet cuff closer to the head is then inflated and the rubber bandage is removed. The arm or leg is lowered and local anaesthetic is injected through the intravenous cannula. After at least five minutes, the lower tourniquet cuff is inflated. Once this has been secured, the upper cuff is released. This sequence ensures that the patient does not feel any pain from the tourniquet, which must remain inflated for at least 45 minutes. If the tourniquet is released prematurely, there is an increased chance that the local anaesthetic will rush through the patient's blood vessels to the heart and brain. The effect on the heart would be to decrease the heart rate and blood pressure. The effect on the brain might be to cause seizures or loss of consciousness.

MONITORED ANAESTHESIA CARE

In many hospitals, anaesthetists provide care to patients having surgical procedures under local anaesthesia only, for example examination of the bladder (cystoscopy). The anaesthetist is available to monitor the patient and to provide intravenous or inhaled anaesthetic agents for additional sedation or pain relief. In the past, this type of care was often termed stand-by (because the anaesthetist was standing by, ready to intervene if necessary). This approach to patient care is now commonly referred to as 'monitored anaesthesia care'.

Because the anaesthetist is caring for the patient, the surgeon is able to focus on the operation, rather than having attention divided between the surgical field and the condition of the patient. For example, should a patient become distressed during the course of the operation, or suffer a complication from the procedure or the local anaesthetic, the anaesthetist provides necessary comfort or resuscitation and the surgeon can continue (if appropriate) with the procedure. One operation occasionally performed under 'local by surgeon' (or monitored anaesthesia care) is that of cataract extraction.

LOCAL ANAESTHESIA

Local anaesthesia refers to the administration of local anaesthetic agents under the skin (subcutaneously). When booked this way on the Operating Room schedule, this technique implies that the surgeon will give the drugs without any involvement of an anaesthetist.

LILY

It is five days before the first signs of labour begin and Lily's waters break, fortunately without any sign of blood. As promised, Tom brings Lily directly to the labour ward. Lily and Tom have re-read the pamphlet that Dr Jenkins gave them and they have talked several times about what Lily would like to do. Tom has said that he will help Lily in whatever way he can, and that if she wants to have anything for pain relief during labour, then that is her choice. Lily decides that she will have an epidural.

When they arrive in the labour ward, Dr Jenkins is again on duty. Lily and Tom speak with her and Lily says that she wants to have an epidural. By now, Lily's contractions have started and are quite regular, every three minutes. Dr Jenkins suggests that the epidural can be inserted now, before the contractions grow stronger and Lily finds it harder to lie still during the procedure. Lily agrees.

Dr Jenkins first inserts a very large intravenous cannula into a vein in Lily's right forearm—because Lily is left-handed—and away from her wrist so that Lily is free to use the arm. Then, with Lily sitting with her back near the edge of the bed, Dr Jenkins inserts an epidural catheter.

By this time the contractions are getting stronger. And although she tries the nitrous oxide, breathing from the mask, Lily begins to wonder how the pain could ever get worse.

Dr Jenkins decides that, because an emergency Caesarean is still a possibility, a plain epidural would be the best option. After the first dose of anaesthetic is injected through the tubing, Dr Jenkins tapes the epidural catheter up Lily's back. Lily is then allowed to lie down, but with a pillow under her left hip. This is to ensure that the weight of the baby in the uterus does not obstruct the flow of blood in the vena cava, the large vein in Lily's abdomen. If this were to happen, Lily might feel faint or the baby might show signs of lack of oxygen.

'Nothing's happened yet!' says Lily, a little distressed, but shortly after, her legs become warm and the pains gradually disappear. However, she is still able to sense when she has a contraction. 'Thank you, Dr Jenkins,' smiles Lily, 'I'm going to enjoy this.'

MATTHEW

On entering the Operating Room, Matthew is asked to sit on the operating table, with his feet over the edge and resting on a high metal stool. The assistant attaches all the necessary monitors and helps Dr Allen to start an intravenous line. Dr Allen then asks the assistant to wrap a warm sheet around Matthew's shoulders and to support Matthew in bending over.

To Matthew he says, 'I'd like you to stay nice and still while I scrub up. It will only take a few minutes.'

Having done so, Dr Allen prepares the area on Matthew's back where the needle will be inserted. He then takes a very fine needle and places it through the skin in the middle of Matthew's lower back.

'You should feel only a slight pin-prick and then a bit of dull pushing.'

Matthew grunts in response.

'That's fine. Now, hold very still while I inject the drug mixture. Is that okay?'

'Yes,' says Matthew in a quiet voice.

'Good, all done,' says Dr Allen. 'Now we'll just have you sit there for a minute, to get most of the drug around your bottom.'

Matthew notices that his feet and legs become warm and then very heavy.

Just then, Dr Allen says, 'Right, we'll have you lie back down on the operating table.'

NICOLA

Dr Solomon picks Nicola up from her mother's arms and cradles her in his own. He then invites Nicola's mother to give her a kiss on the forehead.

Nicola's mum tearfully clutches one of her daughter's tiny hands and asks, 'She will be all right, won't she?'

'She will be fine. I will take very good care of her and I'll come back and see you as soon as it's all over.'

Dr Solomon takes Nicola off to the Operating Room, which he has previously prepared. In Nicola's case, he does not use the separate Anaesthetic Induction Room, so that everything he needs is at hand in the Operating Room. In addition, the temperature of the Operating Room has been turned up so it is very warm, almost tropical.

The operating table's hard mattress is covered with a sheet over a layer of soft sponge. Dr Solomon places Nicola carefully on her back and asks his assistant to steady her with a hand. Overhead is an infrared radiant heater to keep her warm. The assistant peels off the plastic dressing which covers the backs of both of Nicola's hands, wipes away the cream, and applies a tiny wrap-around sensor to Nicola's left thumb. Soon after connecting this to the lead on the anaesthetic monitoring system, a rapid beep-beep is heard and the figures '96' and '142' appear on the screen. These numbers indicate that Nicola's oxygen saturation is 96 per cent and her heart rate is 142 beats per minute.

Dr Solomon nods approvingly. 'Good. Now for the IV. Is everything ready?'

His assistant grasps Nicola's right arm firmly but gently. Dr Solomon takes a tiny intravenous cannula and inserts it into a vein on the back of Nicola's hand. There is a small drop of blood at the end of the cannula where Dr Solomon attaches a connector to the cannula. He asks his assistant—who hardly needs prompting—to secure the cannula with adhesive tape.

Dr Solomon then switches on a flow of oxygen into the anaesthetic circuit, checks the attachment of the mask, and reassures himself that the other equipment is ready. He picks up three syringes—one with an induction drug, one with a muscle relaxant, and one with sterile saline (with which to flush the other two into the intravenous line). He injects the drugs and over the next few minutes he proceeds with unhurried intensity to take over Nicola's breathing, insert an endotracheal tube, and introduce a small needle at the base of her back to inject local anaesthetic. All the time, Dr Solomon watches and listens, alert to any signs that might require any urgent attention.

Once this is done, the equipment is rechecked. Dr Solomon listens with his stethoscope to both of Nicola's lungs, and his assistant then covers Nicola with a reflective blanket.

'We're ready,' says Dr Solomon to the surgeon who is standing patiently, gowned and gloved.

The surgeon proceeds to wash both Nicola's groins with an antiseptic solution.

'That was quick,' he murmurs, nodding toward the clock. 'Seventeen minutes by my reckoning and no hiccups—nice to work with you.'

RICHARD

On the morning of his operation, after a shower, the nurses dress Richard in a hospital gown—neither modest nor warm but very traditional. Soon an orderly from the Operating Room arrives with a trolley and Richard makes himself as comfortable as he can on a narrow, hard conveyance with the mind of a supermarket trolley.

In the Operating Room, a nurse checks Richard's charts and his name-bands and asks on which side he is having his operation. She notes that the surgeon, who visited Richard the previous evening, has used a marker to place a large indelible arrow on the skin over Richard's right hip and that the leg has also been painted by the ward nurse with orange antiseptic solution.

Dr McKenzie arrives, shakes Richard's hand and proceeds to wheel him into the Operating Room. With the help of an assistant, Dr McKenzie gets Richard to lie on his back on the operating table. The assistant starts to attach some monitors—ECG adhesive electrodes, a blood pressure cuff on the left arm, and the pulse oximeter on the left thumb. Meanwhile, Dr McKenzie attaches a soft rubber tourniquet to Richard's right arm to make the veins stand out, injects a small amount of local anaesthetic into the skin on the back of Richard's right hand, and then inserts a large intravenous cannula. Once this is in, Dr McKenzie's assistant hands him a bag of clear intravenous solution attached to clear plastic tubing that is then locked onto the cannula. The assistant adjusts the flow of fluid to a steady trickle. The fluid feels a little cold.

Dr McKenzie then asks Richard to lie on his right side and the assistant helps him to tuck his knees up as high as they can go. Richard has a bit of difficulty raising the right one.

'That's why I'm having this operation,' he quips.

After having checked Richard's position, Dr McKenzie removes the gloves he wore to start the intravenous and goes out of the room to scrub his hands. The assistant has covered as much of Richard as he can, while leaving his back exposed. He asks Richard if he has brought a Walkman or if he would be happy with the surgeon's choice of music.

'Hope you like country and western!'

A few minutes later, Dr McKenzie re-enters the Operating Room holding his wet arms and hands out in front of him with the arms bent up. Water drips from his elbows. The nurse, who is scrubbed, hands him a sterile towel with which he dries his arms. She then gives him a pair of sterile gloves, which he expertly dons. He walks over behind Richard, saying that he will explain everything he does and will tell him before each step. He proceeds to do so, first washing Richard's back with antiseptic, then positioning sterile towels over and around Richard's back, and then inserting the epidural. After this is well positioned and taped in securely, Dr McKenzie and his assistant help Richard to lie on his back again.

Over the next ten minutes, Richard notices that his feet and legs feel warm and heavy and then just seem to disappear as the epidural takes effect. Dr McKenzie asks Richard how he feels.

'Fine, although I can't feel my legs any more.'

'Good. Then I'll just test how high the block is.' He takes a small square of cotton, dips it into some alcohol solution, and then strokes the sponge on Richard's right shoulder. 'Just tell me when you can't feel this as cold,' instructs Dr McKenzie. He gradually works down Richard's chest until there is a noticeable change in sensation just at the belly button.

'Didn't even feel you touch there.'

'Great,' says Dr McKenzie. 'We're ready to get everything set up.' To his assistant he says, 'You can ask the surgeon if he'd like to come down now and scrub.'

Dr McKenzie then injects something into Richard's intravenous line and the rest is just a vague blur.

SUSAN

Dr Wong greets Susan in the Operating Suite waiting room. She has walked there with Eric and a nurse and has already had her injection of subcutaneous heparin to help prevent blood clots forming in the veins of her legs.

'Hi! How are you feeling, Susan?'

'A bit nervous, I can tell you,' Susan replies, holding Eric's hand tightly.

'If you want to say your good-byes, I'm all ready to go. We'll walk to the Operating Room when you're ready.'

They enter the Operating Room together and Susan is surprised by the number of people there. She immediately recognises her surgeon who is talking to a colleague. He comes over to her.

'Hello, Susan. All ready for the big day? Can I introduce my assistant surgeon, Dr Jacobs? She's going to help out. I'll leave you in Dr Wong's care now, and I'll see you and Eric later.'

There are two nurses, already in sterile gowns and gloves, setting out a huge array of shining metal objects. They look up from their work as Dr Wong asks Susan to climb onto the operating table. He introduces the anaesthetic technician, Ben, who steadies Susan as she steps onto a stool and then turns and lies down on the table. Ben places a pillow under her head as she does so and then covers her with a blanket. It feels nice and warm, as if it has been in a heater.

Dr Wong attaches a pulse oximeter probe on her left index finger while Ben fits a blood pressure cuff to her right arm. She feels the cuff suddenly get tight and then gradually release. Some beeping appears on the machine near her head. She is conscious of a large object and some flashing lights. Ben attaches three sticky pads with wires connected, one to each of her shoulders and one to her left hip.

'Just attaching you to the ECG monitor,' says Ben, 'so we can watch your heart rhythm.'

Susan looks up at the huge light suspended above the operating table and wonders how bright it must be when turned on.

'Now, first the IV,' says Dr Wong as Ben takes Susan's left arm and places a tourniquet around it just above the elbow.

'There'll be just a little jab—a bit like the one you already had this morning for the heparin.'

Susan winces a little as Dr Wong injects a tiny amount of local anaesthetic into the skin on her forearm. He then takes a much larger needle and cannula and places it into a vein. Ben releases the tourniquet and connects the intravenous line, allowing some of the fluid to drip into Susan's veins.

'Still okay there?' asks Dr Wong.

'Yes, still here,' says Susan, who manages a faint smile.

'Right, everything ready, Ben?'

Ben nods.

'Now Susan, I'm going to inject some drugs through the intravenous line. You'll feel cold going up your arm and then perhaps a funny taste in your mouth. The next thing you'll know, the operation will be all over. You can count if you like.'

'One ... two ... three ...' Susan slips into unconsciousness as she reaches 'ten'. Dr Wong gently lifts her chin up, allowing her to breathe without snoring, and places a mask over her nose and mouth. As she stops breathing, he takes over, squeezing the bag attached to the circuit and inflating her lungs with oxygen. He then turns on the nitrous oxide and a small amount of isoflurane. About two minutes later, he turns off the nitrous and isoflurane and removes the mask from Susan's face. With the gloved fingers of his right hand, he opens her mouth and then, using his left hand, inserts the metal laryngoscope into the back of her throat. He pulls up on the 'scope, being careful not to touch Susan's top front teeth with it. He peers into the back of her throat.

'Looks as if I might need the introducer,' he murmurs to Ben. 'Can only see the tip of the *epiglottis*.'

Dr Wong removes the 'scope, turns the nitrous and isoflurane back on, and replaces the mask over Susan's face. He continues to ventilate her as he waits for Ben to insert the special length of flexible wire into the breathing tube. Ben then proceeds to bend the end of the tube into the shape of a hockey stick. He holds it up for Dr Wong to see.

'Okay?'

'Great, thanks. Now let's have a go.'

Dr Wong then proceeds to reintroduce the 'scope and then pulls hard on it, so that Susan's head is slightly lifted from the pillow. He takes the tube in his right hand and inserts it into Susan's larynx and down into her trachea.

'In.'

He removes the 'scope carefully, continuing to hold the tube with his right hand. Ben connects the tube to the circuit from which he has detached the mask. They both turn to look at the carbon dioxide monitor. Satisfied that the tube is indeed in the trachea, Dr Wong hits the button on the automatic blood pressure machine and proceeds to inject some more narcotic into the intravenous line.

'Think you could start,' he says to the surgeon, who has been waiting patiently.

'No rush,' replies the surgeon. 'Wouldn't want there to be any problems.'

'Couldn't agree more, but she's going to have a sore throat postop.'

TOBY

Just after ten o'clock, the nurse comes to tell Toby and his parents that it's time to proceed to the Operating Room.

'Can I take my Gameboy?' Toby asks.

'Of course,' is the reply, 'and your teddy bear.'

The four of them, Toby in his pyjamas and slippers, walk to the lift for the journey up three floors to the Operating Suite. There they are met by another nurse, who checks certain details on a form, including items from the chart and Toby's name-band, before the ward nurse returns to the ward. Everyone here is dressed in pale blue pyjama suits. Some have brightly coloured hats, while others are wearing what look like shower caps. Toby is shown a trolley with sheets, a blanket, and a pillow.

'This is your trolley, Toby,' says the nurse. 'You don't have to get on it yet—there are some toys over there, plenty of books to look at, or Nintendo to play with.'

Toby doesn't need to be encouraged. He heads straight for the controller and challenges his father to a car race. Alan reluctantly accepts the challenge, knowing he will be beaten.

Soon, Dr Hansen appears. Her hat is covered with green frogs, and she sees Toby and Alan intently watching the television screen.

'Come on, Toby, time to go,' says Jenny.

'Oh, not yet,' replies Toby, contorting his body as the racing car veers from side to side on the screen.

Alan solves the problem by conceding defeat and Toby, with a small victor's smile, agrees to climb onto the trolley. He kisses Alan and holds his mum's hand while Dr Hansen and her assistant wheel the trolley down the corridor and into a small room.

'This is the sleep room, Toby,' says Dr Hansen. 'Peter, here, is my assistant and he's going to wipe that cream off your hands. Then he will put a special clothes-peg on your finger to tell us what your pulse is. It will start to go "beep-beep" soon.'

Sure enough, a high-pitched beep begins and Toby turns to look at the monitor with all its squiggly lines.

Toby's mother stands by one side of the trolley, holding his hand, while Peter takes his other arm and squeezes it gently below the elbow. Dr Hansen takes Toby's hand and taps it gently on the area where the cream has been, saying how good Toby was and asking if he has a name for his teddy bear or is it just Teddy.

'You'll feel a little push, Toby,' says Dr Hansen as she takes a very fine cannula and needle and proceeds to insert it through the skin and into a vein on the back of Toby's hand.

He gives a little flinch as the needle enters, but otherwise shows no reaction.

'There, that's all done,' says Dr Hansen. 'That was okay, wasn't it? No more needles. And now I'm going to give you some special sleeping medicine. How does that feel? Sometimes it's a bit cold and then you might get a funny taste, but in just a few seconds you'll be asleep and when you wake up you'll have a bit of a sore throat.'

Very quickly Toby begins to stare blankly into space, his eyes wide open. Although the sudden change in Toby's appearance might be frightening to someone not used to it, Jenny knows what to expect. She is also comforted by the smooth manner in which Dr Hansen takes hold of the mask, places it over Toby's face, and adjusts some gas controls on the equipment by her side.

'You can give him a kiss and then nurse will show you the way out,' says Dr Hansen.

'I'm just amazed at how quick it is,' says Jenny, as she leans over and kisses Toby on the part of his cheek not covered by the face mask. 'Look after him, won't you?'

'We'll take good care of him,' replies Dr Hansen.

Chapter 8

After your anaesthetic

After your operation or procedure, you are taken to one of several places. Most commonly, this is the Recovery Room (RR) where there are a number of other patients (depending on the size of the facility) also recovering from their anaesthetics. Other names for this area include the Post-Anaesthetic Recovery Room (PARR) or the Post-Anaesthetic Care Unit (PACU).

If you have undergone a very minor procedure, usually not involving an operation, and in a small surgical clinic or X-ray facility, you may be taken to a recovery 'bay' or place for a single patient. Your care should be the same as you would receive in a Recovery Room.

If you have only a local anaesthetic or monitored anaesthesia care, you might be discharged directly to the day-care ward—for example, after cataract surgery under nerve block. Either your surgeon (in the case of local anaesthesia) or your anaesthetist makes this decision, on the basis of your being stable after the procedure and well recovered from any drugs that you have received.

If you were very ill before surgery, or you had major or complicated surgery (for example, open heart surgery), or complications arose during the course of anaesthesia or surgery, then you might be transferred to an Intensive Care Unit (sometimes known as Intensive Therapy Unit) or High Dependency Unit. (These units are often referred to by their initials: ICU, ITU or HDU.) They offer a more highly specialised level of nursing and medical care.

When you are transferred to the Recovery Room, your anaesthetist provides the Recovery Room nurse with a brief report. This includes a description of:

• your preoperative condition, including any illnesses and medications

- the surgical procedure
- the course of the anaesthetic, including any problems with
  your airway, any need for airway control in the Recovery
  Room, and the adequacy of recovery of muscle strength
- intravenous cannulae
- intraoperative fluid balance (how much intravenous fluid you
  were given and how much fluid you lost, including blood
  loss)
- any other important information.

While this description is being given, the nurse usually places
an oxygen mask over your face to give you extra oxygen, and
attaches a blood pressure cuff and a pulse oximeter. You may or
may not be conscious at this stage. If you are not, then you are
probably positioned on your side, which may become a little
uncomfortable as you awaken. This position, known as the 'coma
position', is commonly used in any situation where a person's ability to protect the airway may be weakened. In this position, the
tongue falls forward, rather than backwards where it may obstruct
breathing. In addition, if the person were to regurgitate or vomit,
the vomitus would drain from the mouth and not be sucked into
the lungs.

You may still have a plastic airway or breathing tube in place.
Exactly when this tube is removed depends in part on your condition and why the tube was inserted, and also on how conscious
you are. Your anaesthetist might choose to remove the tube while
you are still in the Operating Room. If you are still deeply unconscious when you arrive in the Recovery Room, your anaesthetist
might leave the tube in until you 'lighten' or regain consciousness.
(The process of removing the tube is known as *extubation*.) To
many people, the thought of having a breathing tube in place while
awake sounds unpleasant. However, what anaesthetists consider
to be 'awake' in the Recovery Room is not quite the same as being
fully conscious. In fact, being able to open the eyes and mouth and
to take a breath on command are signs that you are probably awake
enough to have the tube removed. Most patients do not remember
any of this.

Once your anaesthetist is assured that your vital signs are stable
and that your safety is assured, the process of 'transfer of care to
the Recovery Room nursing staff' occurs. This means that the

nurses are now responsible for your care and your anaesthetist may leave you to return to the Operating Room to start the anaesthetic for the next patient on the surgical list.

WHO WILL LOOK AFTER ME?

The Recovery Room provides specialised nursing staff who have specific training in the management of common problems of partially anaesthetised patients. Following general anaesthesia, patients in the Recovery Room may develop difficulty breathing. For example, after tonsillectomy there is always the risk of swelling and bleeding from where the tonsils were removed, making it more difficult for patients to breathe. Cardiovascular problems are also of concern. Low blood pressure (hypotension) can occur because of blood loss or from blood pooling in the veins, which dilate as body temperature is restored to normal. High blood pressure (hypertension) may be due to pain, pre-existing hypertension, an increased concentration of carbon dioxide in the blood, or from having a full bladder. Common but less life-threatening problems include pain, nausea, and vomiting. Usually your anaesthetist leaves orders for painkillers or analgesics, drugs to combat nausea and vomiting (anti-emetics), and intravenous fluids. These orders may be written after consultation with your surgeon, but your anaesthetist is the doctor in charge of your care in the Recovery Room.

REGAINING CONSCIOUSNESS

When are you going to start?

This is the question most often asked by patients when they are regaining consciousness in the Recovery Room, although the operation is now over. The reason probably lies in the fact that general anaesthesia is really a state of 'suspended animation'. During this state, many body functions are temporarily changed. One of these functions is that of the 'clock' that all of us carry within us. This clock gives us the ability to know that time has passed. For example, when we awaken in the morning from a normal night's sleep, we usually know that we have slept for some time. With general anaesthesia, this ability to tell that time has

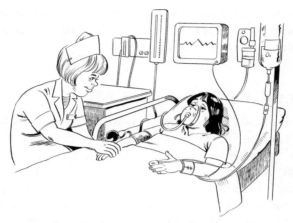

passed seems to be temporarily blocked. We are not sure how or why this happens, but the effect seems to last only as long as the state of unconsciousness.

What will I see?

At first your vision is likely to be somewhat blurred. It is not uncommon to see more than one nurse or anaesthetist, even though only one is present at your bedside! Gradually you will be able to focus better. Although it is reassuring to be able to see clearly, many hospitals do not recommend that you take your glasses with you to the Operating Room. This is because of the risk that they might be mislaid or dropped while you are unconscious. In that case, you would not be able to wear your glasses until you returned to the ward. Some hospitals do allow you to keep your spectacles with you.

If the hospital allows your relatives to be with you in the Recovery Room, it may be best to leave your spectacles with them. (Some hospitals do not allow any visitors in the Recovery Room.) If your child normally wears glasses, it is a good idea to have them available, so that the Recovery Room nurse can give them to your child as he or she awakens.

What will I hear?

In general, your hearing is not significantly affected, although you may well forget instructions that are given to you during the early recovery period. Some people complain that sounds are louder than normal, but this is usually only temporary and is due to complex interactions between the various anaesthetic drugs and your hearing mechanism. A few patients develop sudden loss of hearing in one or both ears after an anaesthetic and operation. One reason for this problem is the effect of pressure from the nitrous oxide on the eardrum and Eustachian tube (inside the ear). These patients may complain of pain and/or clicking and popping in the ear, like that which occurs in an aeroplane when climbing or descending. Very rarely, the mechanism of the hearing loss cannot be explained and hearing may or may not recover. However, it must be emphasised that this complication is extremely uncommon.

If you normally wear a hearing aid, you may choose to leave it in during the operation. This can be helpful if you have significant hearing loss and are having your operation under regional anaesthesia, when you might need to hear what your anaesthetist is saying to you. Other patients might choose not to wear their aids, especially if they fit loosely and do not provide good hearing. Some patients prefer not to hear anything that goes on in the Operating Room or the Recovery Room and therefore leave the aids at their bedside.

What will I say?

You may say all sorts of things, mostly related to your sense of *disorientation* or your surprise at being awake so soon. You may refer to pain or other discomfort, which can then be treated appropriately. Occasionally, patients say suggestive things to their medical or nursing staff, because the effect of the drugs is to temporarily remove some inhibitions. This is very uncommon, and if it does occur, it is always treated with discretion. This type of reaction lasts only a brief time and patients have no memory of the event. If relatives are present, they should not be concerned.

Will I be in pain?

Your anaesthetist endeavours to ensure that you are as pain-free as possible at the end of your operation or procedure. This is not always easy to achieve. Some of the anaesthetic drugs provide some pain relief, but need to be stopped at the end of the anaesthetic so that you regain consciousness. A number of techniques are used to control postoperative pain, most being started during the anaesthetic. These techniques can be modified as necessary in the early postoperative phase in the Recovery Room, so that you have the maximum possible comfort. With some conditions, however, complete obliteration of pain may not be possible without risk of complications, especially where control of breathing may be affected.

Will I feel sick?

You may feel nauseated and it is not uncommon for patients to vomit or dry retch once or twice in the Recovery Room. Often this brings up some mucus or bile-stained fluid, and is usually the only time that vomiting occurs, although some nausea may continue. Your anaesthetist may have given you some anti-emetic drugs during the anaesthetic if vomiting is thought likely to be a problem. Even if an anti-emetic has not already been given, it is not too late to administer some in the Recovery Room, and the nurse will arrange for it to be given.

Will I be cold?

You may feel cold, and shivering is not uncommon in the Recovery Room. This is due partly to the fact that anaesthesia decreases the body's ability to maintain a normal temperature, resulting in loss of body heat. Shivering is also due to some of the anaesthetic drugs that 'switch on' the shivering mechanism in the recovery phase.

In recent years, much more attention has been paid to ensuring maintenance of body heat during surgery and so postoperative shivering is now less common. Devices such as warm water mattresses, warm air blankets, insulation wraps, and warmers for intravenous fluids and anaesthetic gases have contributed to this improvement. Some hospitals suggest that patients wear warm socks during the operation.

CHILDREN IN THE RECOVERY ROOM

Children often go through a period of disorientation and restlessness that may be difficult to manage for a short time as they regain consciousness. This affects younger children more frequently and is quite normal, although distressing to parents or guardians. The reaction is more common after short procedures where there is minimal use of narcotic painkillers or other sedatives. The restlessness may be prevented or treated by the use of sedatives, either at the time or given as premedication. However, the effect of any of these drugs is to prolong recovery time significantly. If this type of distress has been a concern on previous occasions or with siblings, you should discuss the management with your child's anaesthetist.

Children are frequently able to drink while still in the Recovery Room. Usually babies can be breast-fed, unless there is some particular reason to not do so.

In most modern surgical suites it is usual to allow parents to sit with their children as they awaken from anaesthesia. You may be encouraged to do so, once the nurse caring for your child is satisfied that all vital signs are stable and recovery is proceeding normally. You should ask your hospital or anaesthetist whether they allow this practice.

Some young children do not wake easily after an anaesthetic, especially if the anaesthetic coincides with the child's normal sleep pattern. This is more likely if the recovery phase coincides with the child's usual bedtime and if the child is normally a heavy sleeper. The situation may be disturbing to parents, but is quite normal. The use of painful stimulation to 'wake the child up' is discouraged.

DISCHARGE FROM THE RECOVERY ROOM

Anaesthetists and nurses use specific criteria to determine if a patient is fit enough to be discharged from the Recovery Room. A patient must:

- be able to breathe properly without assistance
- have stable vital signs (for example, blood pressure and heart rate)
- be awake (except children, as discussed above) and orientated
- have minimal pain and nausea.

If there is any bleeding from the surgical site, it should be well controlled and minimal.

If a patient meets all these criteria, generally the nurse may discharge the patient from the Recovery Room without the anaesthetist being present. However, some patients require review by their anaesthetist, even if they meet the discharge criteria. Other patients might not meet the criteria, despite having spent what appears to be an appropriate length of time in the Recovery Room. This might be because of complications from the operation or anaesthetic, or from problems with pre-existing conditions. These patients might require further consultation (e.g. by a cardiologist) or referral to an HDU or ICU.

The nurses are responsible for maintaining a record of the patient's condition in the Recovery Room. They are also responsible for conveying relevant information to the ward, unit, or clinic to which the patient is to be transferred. Depending on the operation, most patients stay for a minimum of 30 minutes in the Recovery Room, although this time may be increased to a few hours if the patient has undergone a very complex operation. Occasionally patients have to stay in the Recovery Room although they are ready for discharge because of administrative problems within the hospital, such as a lack of nurses or porters to transport the patient, or a lack of beds on the ward.

Toby

Toby arrives in the Recovery Room. He is lying on his side on the trolley. There is a little blood and mucus around his mouth and a trickle of blood from one nostril onto an absorbent pad. Dr Hansen is supporting Toby's jaw and checking his breathing all the way down the corridor from the Operating Room.

The nurse who will be looking after Toby takes the oximeter and places it on Toby's finger, to monitor his pulse and oxygen again. Toby's teddy is tucked under his arm.

Dr Hansen and the surgeon both speak briefly to Alan and Jenny, who are sitting in the waiting room.

'Everything is fine. Toby is in the Recovery Room, still sleeping. You'll be able to be with him shortly. The nurse will give you a call.' A few minutes later, they are called to the Recovery Room to be with Toby as he wakes up. He begins to get quite restless and tries to get up on all fours. Jenny rushes to the end of the trolley to reassure him.

The nurse explains that children often go through a period of restlessness as they wake up from anaesthesia. 'It's because they're half asleep and half awake—disoriented in a strange environment. Sometimes they get quite upset, but it usually doesn't last too long.'

After about 15 minutes, Toby settles back to a comfortable doze. A few minutes later he opens his eyes and complains that his throat is a little sore, and asks if he can have a drink. The nurse offers him a sip of water from a paper cup.

Dr Hansen returns to the Recovery Room with the next patient who has also had a tonsillectomy. She asks Toby and his parents if everything is okay.

'He was a bit restless for a while,' says Alan, 'but he didn't seem to be too uncomfortable and Nurse explained that kids are often a bit out of sorts as they first wake up.'

'Yes,' says Dr Hansen. 'It's just that they're not sure of their surroundings and you know how some kids wake up grumpy in the morning—I've got three of them and they're all like that!'

Alan nods understandingly.

BACK ON THE WARD

After discharge from the Recovery Room, you are transported to a ward. This may be a regular ward, where you will spend at least one night. The length of time you spend in the hospital ward varies according to the severity and length of your operation, and to a certain extent the complexity of anaesthesia.

Alternatively, you may be taken to a day ward, where you spend only a few hours before going home. Many procedures (up to 70 per cent in some countries) are now performed on a day-stay basis, with the patient staying in the hospital or clinic for less than 24 hours. Not all procedures are suitable for discharge home so soon, especially major operations involving surgery on the brain or within the chest or abdominal cavities, or surgery requiring continuous intravenous or epidural pain relief, such as after total hip replacement.

No matter how long you stay, the nurses will ensure that you are continuing to follow the expected course of recovery from your anaesthetic and operation.

Relief of postoperative pain

The management of postoperative pain is a continuation of the pain control provided during your anaesthetic. Both your anaesthetist and your surgeon may be involved in prescribing the drugs used for relieving your pain.

There are several options for postoperative pain control, which can be divided into the route or manner by which these drugs are given. These options include the following.

Oral or rectal analgesics and anti-inflammatory drugs

These drugs include paracetamol or acetaminophen (alone and with codeine), codeine phosphate, anileridine, pethidine, buprenorphine, indomethacin, and ketorolac. Most of them are taken as tablets, although a syrup may be used for children. Many of these drugs may also be given as suppositories. They are used for mild to moderate pain and are suitable for patients who are staying in hospital after minor operations or who are to be discharged home the day of the operation. These drugs have few common side-effects, apart from constipation with codeine and the risk of reduced breathing if an overdose of pethidine or anileridine is taken. There have been a few rare cases of sudden onset of kidney failure in patients who have been given ketorolac, although the evidence proving such a link is not clear.

Intramuscular injections

Most often this route is used for the administration of narcotic analgesics. These are given on an intermittent basis, usually every few hours. A typical order would be 'morphine 10 mg im q4h prn' (which translates to 'give 10 milligrams of morphine intramuscularly every four hours—but no sooner—if the patient wishes it'). This technique provides adequate, but not very good, pain control. Shortly after receiving the injection, the patient gets the effect of a large amount of narcotic, which may reduce breathing and produce sedation and even confusion. Then the effect of the drug wears off, leaving the patient in pain until the next injection. The use of intramuscular injections is declining in popularity, not only because continuous administration methods provide better pain control, but also because of the discomfort of the injection.

Continuous intravenous infusion

With this technique, narcotics are delivered directly via an intravenous cannula at a predetermined rate. This provides a steady concentration of drug in the bloodstream (in contrast to the intramuscular technique, which gives a variable blood concentration). Nursing or medical staff may adjust the rate of infusion, according to the pain relief obtained.

Continuous subcutaneous infusion of narcotic analgesics

This is similar to the intravenous method, except that the fluid is pumped through a fine needle into the tissues just under the skin, usually on the abdomen. Because the volume of fluid is small, there is little swelling or discomfort and the drug is well absorbed.

Patient-controlled analgesia (PCA)

This is another method of intravenous injection of narcotics, except that the patient controls the analgesia by pushing a button to determine when the injection is given. The administration of the drug is determined by a pump that has been programmed to deliver a fixed, safe dose of drug every time the patient requests it. There is a maximum hourly dose and a 'lock-out' interval that can be adjusted to prevent overdose. (This is similar to bank machines, which have limits on withdrawals.)

This technique is based on the principle that a patient who has become sleepy will not push the button until the effect of the drug wears off. Of course, this requires that only the patient, and not a friend or family member, pushes the PCA button. Often anaesthetists are in charge of programming these pumps, although surgeons or specially trained nurses may also do so. If necessary, the dose and timing of the drug may be adjusted by reprogramming. Drugs commonly administered by this method include morphine, pethidine (meperidine), and fentanyl. Some doctors also prescribe a constant infusion (a 'background infusion') of a small amount of narcotic, so that there is always some pain relief present. However, this technique carries a greater risk of reduction of breathing than does the 'demand' technique alone, although it is useful in certain patients with extreme pain.

Spinal narcotic injection

Some anaesthetists like to add a small amount of a narcotic when they inject local anaesthetic into the spinal fluid at the time of the operation. This can provide very good pain relief. For example, a woman having a Caesarean section might not need any other pain medication after the operation if she has received some spinal ('intrathecal') narcotic.

Spinal or epidural infusions

Continuous infusions of local anaesthetics and/or narcotic analgesics into the spinal fluid or epidural space may be given for several days after surgery. The advantage with this technique is that there is little sedation, compared with other methods. These methods are particularly useful for patients undergoing chest operations (thoractomies) or upper abdominal operations, or major orthopaedic surgery to the hips and legs. These operations are painful and most patients require large amounts of intramuscular narcotics to provide adequate pain relief, with the possible risk of reduced breathing. Use of an epidural or spinal means that the patient can actually be pain-free.

Nerve blocks

In addition to general anaesthesia, some anaesthetists like to perform a nerve block—to provide analgesia (pain relief) of the area in which the operation or procedure is to take place. This is commonly done for children undergoing circumcision (with a penile nerve block) or hernia repair (with a caudal anaesthetic). Some anaesthetists believe that blocking pain nerves before the patient has any pain actually decreases the amount of pain relief required. This is termed 'pre-emptive analgesia'.

General pain management

Two other important points must be made about pain management. The first is the role of the Acute Pain Service (APS). In the 1970s, researchers began to investigate different methods for the relief of postoperative pain. Then in the 1980s, anaesthetists started to apply this knowledge to improve provision of pain relief. These methods included all those described above. Use of these different techniques has varied widely between institutions; however, most large anaesthetic departments provide a postoperative analgesia service (or Acute Pain Service). Successful programs rely on the assistance of dedicated, specially trained nursing support.

The other important point about pain management is that all patients who receive narcotics are at risk of reduced breathing. Some patients need to be looked after in special care units, not only because of the narcotics but for other medical or surgical reasons. Other patients require frequent monitoring, but can be cared for with regular nursing.

How bad is your pain?

Regular assessment is made of your pain after surgery, but you should tell your treating doctors and nurses if your pain is not controlled. In many hospitals, a scoring system is used to assess the effectiveness of pain treatment. The scoring system usually asks you to score the severity of pain on a scale of zero to ten, with zero being no pain and ten being unbearable pain.

Am I likely to become addicted to narcotics?

No, the administration of narcotic drugs after surgery, to provide relief of surgical pain, does not lead to addiction, even when large doses are required.

Are there other methods of pain relief?

There are other methods of pain relief that do not involve the administration of drugs. These 'non-pharmacological' methods include:

- **Application of warmth:** Heated gel or beanbag pads may be used, as may infrared lamps. Great care must be taken to avoid burning the skin, especially in the elderly and those with fragile skin or poor circulation. Lamps, in particular, should only be used for a short time.
- **Distraction:** This method of pain relief is useful in patients of all ages, but particularly in children. The idea is to concentrate the mind on something other than the pain. This can be done by reading, doing puzzles, story-telling, looking out a window at a busy street, and even watching television.
- **Relaxation:** Three ways of relaxing and reducing the psychological awareness of pain are listening to music, meditating, and having a massage.

Dealing with nausea and vomiting

Postoperative nausea and vomiting (PONV) is one of the most common postoperative complications, affecting as many as 40 per cent of patients. The patient most likely to vomit is a young, non-smoking, overweight woman who has undergone gynaecological surgery. Also at risk are patients with a history of PONV and those with a history of motion sickness (in a car or aeroplane or at sea).

All anaesthetic agents have been blamed, with narcotics often implicated. Indeed, the anaesthetic is most often blamed for all PONV, even when nausea and vomiting occur days after the operation and all traces of the anaesthetic have disappeared from the body.

Other factors may contribute, including:

- preoperative conditions, such as vomiting, increased pressure in the brain, intoxication with alcohol or other drugs
- operations on the eyes, the inner ear, the testicles, or tonsils
- postoperative conditions, such as the presence of blood in the stomach (which no anti-emetic can counter) or blockage of the bowel
- pain and anxiety
- the presence of other vomiting patients or the smell of food
- rapid movement (as on a stretcher) or even slight elevation of the head from the pillow

- narcotics given during the anaesthetic or in the postoperative period.

Many of these factors can be avoided or treated, to reduce the chance of postoperative nausea and vomiting occurring. Your anaesthetist makes all attempts to ensure that you do not suffer from PONV. However, complete prevention of this complication is not possible.

Disorientation in the elderly

Elderly patients, especially those who are frail, often experience a period of disorientation after an operation, which may last for several days. This disorientation is similar to dementia, where memory appears to be very limited. Family and friends should treat the patient as normally as possible, and be reassured that the condition is probably temporary. The patients themselves have little or no memory of the events which occur during this period, and there is no need to mention it to them once they recover.

JOHN

John is sitting on the edge of his bed, coughing and holding a small plastic bowl which contains some mucus speckled with blood. It is now some six hours since his return to the ward, and he has been coughing on and off for the last two or three. He is wide awake and Mary is rubbing his back, and passing him a glass of water each time he begins coughing.

There is a pulse oximeter sensor on his index finger that keeps falling off with each bout of coughing. Mary replaces it each time, and when everything is calm the monitor reads a saturation of around 95 per cent.

John has a fine plastic tube running under his nose, which is connected to the oxygen outlet near the head of his bed. There are two little prongs, one under each nostril, through which John is receiving some additional oxygen. It's annoying but necessary.

John was quite comfortable and only coughing occasionally when he first returned to the ward, but now the local anaesthetic in his throat has worn off and all those years of smoking are having their effect.

He has a small dressing over a wound at the base of his neck, from the mediastinoscopy. It is not worrying him particularly—certainly not as much as the cough. The nurses suggested a little while ago that he take some codeine, but John refused despite Mary's protestations.

Just then, Dr Williams and the surgeon arrive. They explain that everything went very well and that there doesn't appear to be any obvious involvement of the lymph nodes in his chest. 'But we have to wait on the pathology results,' cautions the surgeon.

'You don't look too comfortable, John. Have you had any pain-killer?' asks Dr Williams.

'No,' answers Mary.

'Well, I think you should have some. I'll get the nurse to give you some codeine.'

'Thanks . . . thanks very much,' says John.

'He'll be right,' says Mary.

Soon after, the nurse arrives with two tablets and John dutifully swallows them. 'Thanks,' he says.

Lily

Lily is sitting in an armchair cradling the new baby. Tom, the proud father, stands alongside.

'I've been on the phone to my mother, and she is very happy that I didn't need an operation,' Lily says. 'It was much better than I thought—I didn't really feel any pain at all, yet I knew what was happening all the time, and I was able to hold Constance as soon as she was born!'

Matthew

Dr Allen knocks on the door and enters. He finds Matthew reclining in bed with his head propped up and a large number of open folders and papers scattered about.

'How are you feeling, Matthew?' he asks.

'Apart from the strange feeling in my legs, I'm fine—really good. Not having any sedation wasn't so bad after all. I've had some afternoon tea and I'm looking forward to dinner—with a nice glass of red!'

'Great. Any problems?'

'Well, I had a bit of trouble having a pee, but that seems to be okay now—no, everything's fine.'

'You're happy to stay until morning?'

'Yes, I've sorted out the office and I've got all my papers here—and there are no phone interruptions! Mind you, I'll be out of here first thing tomorrow!'

'Good. Get the nurses to call me if there is anything worrying you.'

'I will . . . and thank you.'

NICOLA

Dr Solomon hastens to the waiting room, just down the corridor from the operating suite.

'Nicola's fine,' he says to Nicola's mother. 'She's in the Recovery Room and is virtually awake. You'll be able to see her shortly.'

Shortly after, Nicola is joined by her mother and is soon resting in her arms. She appears perfectly comfortable, but before long starts to cry irritably. The nurse asks Nicola's mother if she thinks Nicola is hungry.

'Certainly sounds like it.'

'Do you want to try her at the breast?' asks the nurse.

'Is it okay, so soon?'

'Yes, Nicola will tell us if she's not ready.'

In a few minutes, Nicola is sucking contentedly and her mother smiles, giving a little sigh of relief. 'Isn't she beautiful?' she asks the nurse.

'She's gorgeous.'

RICHARD

It is the second day after the operation and Richard still has his epidural in place. It is connected via a long fine plastic tube to a syringe pump. This machine is steadily pumping a small amount of local anaesthetic and narcotic mixture into his back. He feels comfortable and is eating and drinking, although he doesn't have a great appetite. The day before is a vague blur. Richard had been asking for his wife and making other strange comments, in between appearing to be perfectly normal.

His daughter arrives with a basket of fruit and is pleased to see that he is much better.

'Hello. How are you? Oh, what a wonderful basket of fruit,' says Richard brightly.

'I'm well. How about you?' asks his daughter in return.

'I feel really very good—can't remember much about yesterday—must have had a good sleep. Did you call?'

'Yes, I was here, but you were having a really good rest,' his daughter replies with a hint of a smile.

Dr McKenzie appears at the door not long after. 'You're looking much better today,' he says.

'Am I? I don't remember seeing you yesterday,' replies Richard.

'You weren't quite yourself then, but that's not unusual for someone of your age having a major operation. You just needed a good sleep.'

Dr McKenzie checks the epidural chart with the nurse, noting any changes in dose. He then uses alcohol-soaked cotton wool to map the extent of the block or numbness.

'Excellent. Everything's going well. We'll keep the epidural going for another day and get you onto some tablets for pain before we finally remove the epidural catheter. The nurse will be getting you moving again this afternoon. We held off yesterday and now we don't want those legs to get stiff or develop any clots.'

'I'll be pleased when I'm back in my garden,' says Richard. 'I hope someone's watering it.'

'Don't worry about the garden,' responds his daughter. 'Let's get you on your feet first.'

Susan

Susan has been back on the ward for about three hours and is feeling a little nauseated. Her incision is reasonably comfortable and she has been using the patient-controlled analgesia (PCA) as needed.

'It's not as bad as I thought. The PCA certainly controls most of the pain and I'm able to sleep. In fact, I keep drifting off. But

I've thrown up a couple of times in the last hour and that hurt a bit.'

Dr Wong gave Susan an anti-emetic during the anaesthetic. However, it doesn't seem to have been fully effective.

'And my throat is quite sore. Reckon I should stop talking.'

An hour later, after consulting with Dr Wong over the phone, the nurse injects a different anti-emetic into Susan's intravenous line. Soon Susan is feeling much more comfortable as the nausea fades away. She drifts off again into a light sleep.

TOBY

Toby has his drink of water and is then collected by the ward nurse. On arrival back in the ward, he is transferred to a bed where he curls up, clutching his teddy bear, and promptly goes to sleep.

An hour later he is awake and thirsty. He drinks some cordial and the nurse gives him some painkilling syrup mixed in a little cordial. He says he feels fine and is soon ready for something to eat.

'No McDonald's yet,' says the nurse, 'but what about ice cream?'

Toby nods with a hint of a smile and then lies back to watch the cartoons on television.

HOME

In some centres, hotel-type facilities, with access to nursing and medical staff, provide an intermediate step between hospital care and home care during the early recovery period.

If you have undergone day surgery, you may be discharged from the hospital or clinic only when you are fully conscious and able to walk. Most facilities require that you be accompanied by a responsible adult, who either drives you home or accompanies you in a taxi. This person or another adult should stay with you for the first night.

It is common practice to advise all patients not to drive automobiles, operate equipment, or make important personal or business decisions for at least 24 hours. This is because any residual effects of drugs might interfere with your ability to make decisions. Patients are also routinely advised about the additive effects of alcoholic beverages and sedative drugs.

How do I cope at home afterwards?

Ideally you should have someone (a relative or a friend) stay with you for a period of time after anaesthesia and surgery. One reason for this is because the effects of the operation may limit your physical activity. You may need assistance with everyday things, such as washing and dressing. Even when you are physically quite capable of attending to your own needs, you should arrange to have someone with you, in case you develop pain, vomiting, dizziness, or a surgical problem such as bleeding.

You should be given clear instructions as to what to do in the case of complications, such as pain, bleeding, or persistent vomiting. You should also know when you are to return to see your surgeon.

Coping with pain

Your surgeon or your anaesthetist will give you a prescription for pain-relieving medication. This is normally in the form of tablets or capsules, and may include some anti-inflammatory drugs. (This combination of drugs has been found to be helpful postoperatively.) You should continue to take these until you can resume your normal everyday activity. Failure to use pain-relieving medication when you have pain may restrict your activity and so prolong your recovery period. You should not hesitate to contact your anaesthetist, surgeon, or family doctor if you have any problems.

Coping with cancer pain

Some patients are in constant, severe pain from cancer or another debilitating and chronic disease. These patients can receive considerable relief if their pain is adequately assessed and then managed. Techniques for pain management include:

- non-drug therapies, such as heat, distraction, relaxation
- prescription of adequate doses of appropriate drugs, including narcotics, sedatives, and tranquillisers

- prescription of drugs and other therapies to deal with the side-effects of the painkillers—for example, laxatives for the treatment of constipation from narcotics
- changing how painkillers are given (subcutaneous infusions, implantation of epidural catheters and pumps)
- nerve blocks, which can be either temporary or permanent.

All these techniques can be used at home. However, good follow-up from an anaesthetist or chronic pain doctor is needed.

Vomiting

Nausea and vomiting can normally be controlled by medication. It is unlikely that you will be discharged from hospital if vomiting is a major problem. However, if vomiting becomes troublesome at home, you should contact your anaesthetist, surgeon, or family doctor as soon as possible. Persistent vomiting can be dangerous because you cannot take in the fluids that you need for normal body function. Severe vomiting may put excess strain on healing stitches or staples. There are a number of drugs that are likely to be quite effective.

Eating and drinking

You can eat and drink whatever appeals to you. However, it is sensible to begin by drinking water and then progress to other drinks, such as ginger ale or tea. It is better to avoid milk-based liquids, and to abstain from alcoholic beverages for at least twenty-four hours. Once you are able to tolerate drinking clear liquids, it is probably safe to try eating something light, such as toast or soup.

Can I breast-feed after my anaesthetic?

There is no danger to your baby from any of the drugs that you receive during anaesthetic. Most of them are destroyed or eliminated from the body quite quickly, and the concentrations in breast milk are very small. Even morphine and similar drugs are present in only very tiny amounts.

Driving

You should not drive any vehicle (including riding a bicycle) for at least 24 hours after a general anaesthetic. We do not tolerate people driving with alcohol in their blood. Similarly, you should be certain that all sedative drugs have been eliminated from your body before attempting to drive.

Work

You can return to work when you feel able to do so, as guided by your surgeon and family doctor. From the anaesthetist's point of view, during the first 24 hours you should remain at home. Also within that time you should not drive, operate any machinery, or make any important decisions. After 24 hours you can return to work, although you may feel more tired than normal at the end of the day.

Convalescence

The process of surgical care and hospitalisation no longer involves a stay of days to weeks. Nor does it involve supervised convalescence. Instead, many patients spend only a few hours in a hospital or clinic and then go home. In addition, because of the advances in anaesthetic drugs and techniques, many patients feel quite clear-headed the next day. As a result, there is a temptation to resume all normal activities.

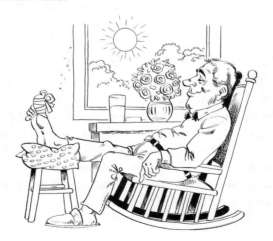

While getting back to normal activity is important, you must also give your body adequate rest and time to recover. As stated earlier, patients do not simply undergo an anaesthetic. They also undergo some kind of operation or procedure. This in itself is stressful, with the body reacting by producing stress hormones. Patients who complain that they were 'exhausted for weeks' after their last anaesthetic are encouraged to think about what they did after their last operation. Most often, these patients then relate that they proceeded with their lives as though nothing much had happened, and they attempted to do everything they did the day before the operation. Both patients and their families should understand that getting better requires rest, nutritious food, and gentle but progressive exercise.

How do I look after someone who has had an anaesthetic?

If you are placed in the position of caring for a relative or friend who has had an anaesthetic, you need to know what to expect and how you can help.

In the hospital, nurses and other staff care for the patient. Your presence is important in hastening recovery from surgery and anaesthesia, by providing a reassuring link with normal life outside the hospital. You can help by talking, holding a hand, or assisting with everyday activities such as eating and washing. The patient is likely to be a little slower to think and react, especially after a long or complex operation and when painkilling medication is being used on a continuous or frequent basis. This requires patience and tolerance on your part.

The patient may vomit. This is never pleasant, either for the patient or for carers. It is best just to clean up and carry on, rather than making a fuss or reacting negatively—it is not the patient's fault!

At all times, if you are uncertain how to manage the situation or if you need explanation, ask the nursing staff.

When you are caring for the patient at home, the same principles apply. Ensure that the bathroom and toilet facilities are easily accessible and that there is someone available to assist if necessary. You might consider giving the patient a bell to ring when needing help. Make sure that the patient has all prescribed medication and painkillers available. Encourage him or her to take the painkillers, rather than endure unnecessary discomfort.

The patient who has had major surgery and anaesthesia is likely to feel a little tired for anything up to several weeks. This is especially so in older patients. Carers need to be aware of this and to be prepared to seek help at any time. Contact should be made with the patient's family doctor as soon as possible after discharge from hospital.

I'm not sure I can look after Gran after her operation

Looking after an elderly relative after discharge from hospital can present major difficulties for families. Recovery from anaesthesia and surgery takes longer than with a young, fit patient. An elderly patient may suffer temporary forgetfulness. This becomes particularly important if there is a need to remember such things as the taking of regular doses of prescription medicine.

Most importantly, elderly patients need to return to their usual level of activity, although this may be a slow process. Lying in bed and sitting in a chair for prolonged periods after surgery puts anyone at risk of developing a blood clot or deep vein thrombosis (DVT) in a vein in the leg or pelvis. Such clots can be potentially lethal if they become dislodged and travel to the heart and lungs where they block the flow of blood.

Special concerns about caring for children after an anaesthetic and operation

Will my child vomit on the way home?

If your child is prone to car or motion sickness, he or she is more likely to vomit during the journey from hospital to home. The chance of vomiting is further increased if the child has already had something to drink or eat and if a dose of narcotic painkiller has been given.

Drugs are available that are very effective in reducing the chance of nausea and vomiting. These drugs are called anti-emetics and may have been given by the anaesthetist while your child was still anaesthetised.

Continued vomiting, particularly by an infant or a small child, requires urgent attention. The excess loss of fluid with lack of intake can rapidly lead to dehydration and severe illness. If you are concerned, contact your anaesthetist or surgeon immediately.

How do I know if my child is in pain?

Children feel pain just as adults do. Similarly, they deserve the same attention to control of pain. In general, children tell things as they are. If it hurts, they say so. They also show other signs in keeping with the severity of the pain—for example, whimpering or crying. Small infants may be difficult to assess as far as pain management is concerned. Crying may be an indication of either pain or hunger, or both. Infants can often be pacified by feeding and they will then sleep peacefully. If they remain unhappy despite having had their normal feed, it is likely that they are in pain. Grimacing and drawing up of the legs may be additional signs.

What can I give my child for pain relief?

The most commonly used painkiller in children is paracetamol (acetaminophen). This drug may be given as a tablet, a suppository, or a liquid (which comes in different flavours). Suppositories are easy to use in small infants and a plastic freezer bag may be used as a substitute for a glove when placing the suppository in the rectum.

Most children are given their first dose of paracetamol (acetaminophen) at the time of surgery and so they may not need any more for a few hours. Your child may have received a general anaesthetic plus a local anaesthetic without any other painkiller. If so then the first dose of paracetamol (acetaminophen) is given before the local anaesthetic wears off. You are told when to do this, as well as which drug and how much.

Stronger analgesics (painkillers) may be required, especially in the first 24 hours after surgery. Codeine is commonly used and is usually given by mouth. Side-effects include constipation and nausea, but these are uncommon with a small number of doses.

Anti-inflammatory analgesic drugs may be used, although not all are approved for use in children. Your anaesthetist will provide details about doses.

Mixtures of drugs may be beneficial, reducing the likelihood of side-effects. Preparations that combine paracetamol (acetaminophen) with codeine are common and some also contain other additives, including mild sedatives.

Aspirin should not be used in children under the age of twelve years. This is because a rare, usually fatal, inflammation of the brain called Reye's syndrome can result when children take aspirin.

When can my child eat and drink?

The simple answer to this question is 'When your child feels like it'. Your child should not be forced to drink something and may not want to drink until after arriving home after day-stay surgery.

Your child should start with sips of water, progressing to ginger ale or cordial, and then to milk. The same applies to eating—begin with easily digested food, such as jelly and bread and butter, although some children like to start with ice cream. It is not unusual, however, for children to want something more substantial; some have been known to enthusiastically consume a hamburger three hours after a tonsillectomy.

Will my child have nightmares?

Sleep disturbance, including nightmares, is frequently described after hospitalisation, surgery and anaesthesia. The less stressful the hospitalisation, the less likely sleep will be disturbed. Things that may reduce the chance of a sleep disturbance include:

- good preparation beforehand (see chapter 5)
- a harmonious family
- the child being accustomed to other carers, such as a babysitter, rather than being overprotected
- parents who are calm, as children can sense parental anxiety
- the presence of one or both parents as much as possible throughout the hospital stay
- sympathetic medical and hospital staff
- needles not being used
- good pain control
- a short stay in the hospital.

When can my child resume full activity?

The answer to this question is again simple: 'When he or she feels like it'. If the operation requires a period of modified activity, your child's surgeon will advise you of this. In general, there are no particular guidelines and you will be surprised at how quickly your child returns to a normal state of activity.

What about swimming?

There may be a surgical reason to recommend against swimming— for example, grommets (tubes) in the ears or a large surgical wound. If not, then swimming should be considered as a part of full activity.

What about returning to school?

Unless there is a surgical reason for delay, your child may return to school as soon as he or she regains full and normal activity. It is wise to inform the teaching staff of the operation. The teachers will then be aware if any untoward reactions do occur, but should otherwise treat your child normally.

Chapter 9

Common fears

People have fears about all sorts of things in life, especially those they don't understand—hence the reason for this book! Many of the fears about anaesthesia come from snippets of incomplete information or from sensationalist press reports. All have a basis in fact, but need to be explained in context and in detail. It is appropriate for you to discuss your concerns about any of these matters with your anaesthetist.

I DON'T LIKE LOSING CONTROL

This is a common fear. Some patients deal with it by choosing to have a regional or local anaesthetic and going without any sedative drugs during the operation or procedure. Other patients who must have a general anaesthetic choose not to have any premed or sedative before the anaesthetic, so that they can remain in control for as long as possible.

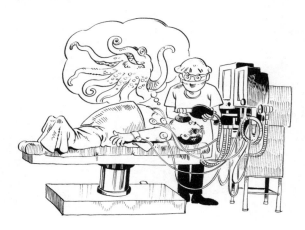

Perhaps the best way of dealing with this fear is to think about why you are concerned. Often patients are afraid that they might say or do things when they are unconscious that would embarrass them. You should be reassured that while you are unconscious you cannot talk or move, and hospital and clinic staff are professionals trained to treat patients with dignity and respect. Some patients are afraid of dying during anaesthesia or of not waking up. However, the chance of something like this occurring as a result of the anaesthetic is very remote.

I'M NOT HAPPY ABOUT HAVING A GENERAL ANAESTHETIC—COULDN'T I JUST HAVE 'TWILIGHT SLEEP'?

'Twilight sleep' is a means of dulling consciousness with sedative and painkilling drugs in order to perform minor procedures. These include removal of skin lesions, sewing up of cuts, examination of the stomach or bowel (endoscopy), and some X-ray procedures where long catheters are inserted into arteries and veins.

Another name for twilight sleep is 'conscious sedation'. The aim of the technique is to give enough sedatives and painkillers so that the patient is calm, but not so much that the patient loses consciousness. The level of consciousness is monitored by the operator or surgeon continuously talking with the patient, who should be conscious enough to respond. If the patient is not able to respond, this indicates that the level of sedation is too deep and there is a risk of problems with breathing.

If the procedure is complex in nature, as with major cosmetic surgery, or if loss of consciousness is likely, then an anaesthetist should be present to care exclusively for the patient. The surgeon or operator is then able to concentrate on the procedure.

COULD I BE ALLERGIC TO ANAESTHESIA?

No, you cannot be 'allergic to anaesthesia' because an anaesthetic may consist of as many as 15 different drugs. Often the phrase 'allergy to anaesthesia' is used to describe a side-effect from the anaesthetic, such as intense nausea, vomiting, agitation, double vision, sore muscles, etc. These are not allergies but exaggerations of some of the common side-effects of anaesthesia or surgery. You should mention these complaints to your anaesthetist, who can take extra measures to try to minimise them.

However, you could be allergic to one of the drugs used as part of an anaesthetic, and the most likely drug to trigger a reaction is a muscle relaxant. Modern muscle relaxants are less likely to do so than previously used drugs.

Local anaesthetics are often blamed. Reactions are possible but are uncommon. Most often, the term 'allergy' has been applied to the fainting reaction seen after a dentist has injected some local anaesthetic. In fact, the reaction is usually a combination of anxiety and the use of adrenaline mixed with the local anaesthetic to make it last longer. This does *not* mean that there has been an allergic reaction to the adrenaline.

Allergies to morphine, pethidine, or other painkillers are commonly described but again, true allergies are rare. Often the term 'allergy' refers to vomiting, which is a common side-effect. (This particular problem is now often preventable, with careful adjustment of dose and the use of anti-emetic drugs.) Blood products and latex rubber (found in much of the equipment in the Operating Room) can also provoke allergic reactions.

Allergies to antibiotics do occur and your anaesthetist needs to know the details of the reactions. Vomiting and abdominal pain are not uncommon side-effects and usually do not mean that you have an allergy. The occurrence of yeast overgrowth or thrush (in the mouth or vagina), fever, and failure of the infection to resolve are also not true allergic reactions.

In general, allergic reactions are rare. Also, it is important to note that allergies to drugs are not passed on in families. Allergic reactions are caused by the presence of antibodies against a specific compound. The existence of antibodies can sometimes be predicted from a patient's previous response—for example, swelling and hives after administration of an antibiotic. Thus, your anaesthetist needs to know about reactions in the past, even though the same drugs will not be used. Very occasionally, an allergic reaction can occur during the anaesthetic, without any previous reaction or warning.

The severity of allergic responses can range from mild (wheeze or rash) to severe (life-threatening *anaphylactic* reactions). As well as anaphylactic or immune-related reactions, some patients develop *anaphylactoid* reactions. Although this type of reaction does not involve antibodies, these reactions may also be severe, through the release of histamine. (Without antibody testing it may be impossible to distinguish between anaphylactoid and anaphylactic reactions.)

If a patient is undergoing a general anaesthetic and is unconscious, the signs of an anaphylactic reaction may vary. The diagnosis is made by the recognition of such things as low blood pressure, wheezing, hives, rash, swelling (oedema) around the eyes or in the mouth and throat, and breathing difficulties.

Anaesthetists are trained to recognise and treat allergic reactions in the Operating Room. However, an important part of treatment of any allergic reaction is prevention. If you have any history of swelling of the face or generalised itching, you should let your anaesthetist know. Skin testing can be used to identify allergens. This may be helpful in identifying the particular drugs causing a reaction in those patients who apparently are 'allergic to anaesthesia'. The prevention of latex allergy includes removing all latex-containing materials from the Operating Room, where possible. Most Operating Rooms have a special kit of equipment for use in caring for latex-allergic patients.

CAN I BE 'IMMUNE' TO THE ANAESTHETIC?

All anaesthetic drugs work when given in the appropriate dose for a patient. However, it must be understood that patients' responses to anaesthetics are different and are related to age, sex, weight, and degree of illness. Your anaesthetist takes all of these factors into account when calculating the doses of drugs you need.

Individuals who have a high intake of alcohol may require larger doses of anaesthetics. This is because the enzymes in the liver that process alcohol and other drugs may be over-active. Patients who are extremely fat usually need more anaesthetic drugs, since the fat acts like a sponge, drawing drugs from the blood and the brain.

DO PATIENTS TALK WHILE THEY ARE UNDER ANAESTHESIA?

It is extremely rare for patients to talk under anaesthesia. Some patients talk a little while losing consciousness. One anaesthetic drug (sodium thiopentone or Pentothal) was popularly known as the 'truth drug' and was used in low doses to extract information. People would talk after being given small quantities of this drug in the same way that some people talk after having a few drinks. However, the dose of Pentothal required to induce anaesthesia is much greater, and the time interval between receiving the drug and becoming deeply unconscious is rarely more than a few seconds.

Patients do not talk during the anaesthetic while they are unconscious, but it is not uncommon for them to do so during emergence from anaesthesia. As we have seen, the first thing most people ask is 'When are you going to start?' Thereafter, the conversation usually relates to the surroundings or to some discomfort, and often there is no memory of this. Occasionally patients swear or talk of other matters that would normally cause some embarrassment to the patient. Nurses who work in the Recovery Room are trained to exercise the utmost discretion at these times.

SHOULD I HAVE AN ENEMA IN CASE?

Uncontrolled emptying of the bowel is uncommon during anaesthesia, except in infants. You do not need to have an enema, or medication to clear out the bowel, unless your surgeon specifically orders one. If so, it is because you are having an operation on or near your bowel.

Uncontrolled emptying of the bladder may occur during anaesthesia but should not happen if you empty your bladder shortly before going to the Operating Room. If you normally take a fluid tablet or diuretic—for example, to control mild high blood pressure—check with your anaesthetist whether or not to take this medication on the morning of the operation. Some anaesthetists believe that it is better not to take a fluid tablet so that their patient is less likely to be troubled by a full bladder either before or after the operation.

Almost all patients receive some intravenous fluids during the anaesthetic and operation. This even applies to patients who are having procedures done under local anaesthesia, such as extraction of a cataract. However, both anaesthetists and surgeons have noticed that it is hard for patients to lie still if they have a full bladder. For this reason, many anaesthetists now try to limit the amount of fluid that cataract patients receive.

Other operations require that patients be given large volumes of intravenous fluid and blood. Often these patients have a catheter inserted into the bladder, usually just after induction of anaesthesia. If the bladder is not emptied, it can contribute to a patient having high blood pressure in the Recovery Room.

COULD MY HEART STOP DURING THE ANAESTHETIC?

Cardiac arrest can and does occur occasionally during anaesthesia, but again, rarely as a result of the anaesthetic. There are multiple causes, including overdose of anaesthetic agents, low blood pressure, and inadequate delivery of oxygen. Rarely, the use of suxamethonium, a muscle relaxant, has been associated with marked slowing of the heart to the point where the patient does not appear to have a heartbeat. This slowing may occur in children as well as in adults. Usually the heart rate rises quickly again, after a drug (atropine) is given to increase it.

One important point must be made. Except for slowing of the heart from suxamethonium, cardiac arrest rarely occurs suddenly. Although a slow heart rate does not reliably indicate that the heart is about to stop, cardiac arrest does not often occur without warning signs. These signs will be detected by the anaesthetist as he or she monitors the patient.

WHAT IF I WAKE UP DURING THE OPERATION?

It is extremely unlikely that you will be awake during a general anaesthetic, but it is possible. There have been descriptions of patients who can recall events that occurred during the operation when they were apparently anaesthetised. This recollection is called *awareness*. Because the depth of consciousness varies, there is a range of what is remembered. The most common memory is brief, vague, and without pain. Some patients have recalled voices or other sounds; a few remember sounds plus touching; and a very, very few have full sensation of the procedure. These patients have been clearly conscious during surgery, unable to move because of the effects of muscle relaxants, and in severe pain.

Certain procedures carry a greater risk of awareness occurring than others. These include Caesarean section (when the amount of anaesthetic is kept purposefully low so as to avoid affecting the baby) and operations for trauma.

However, anaesthetists now recognise that patients may be aware with little outward sign of pain or distress. Although changes in heart rate and blood pressure are two variables used by anaesthetists to alter the depth of an anaesthetic, it is possible for a patient to be aware without any change in these measurements.

Modern anaesthesia demands rigorous attention to the doses of drugs given. Also important is the continuous monitoring of many variables, including aspects of each patient's responses and concentrations of anaesthetic gases inhaled. Some indication of the depth of anaesthesia can now be measured using a recently available monitor—the BIS (Bispectral Index Monitor).

It is hard to differentiate a patient's memories of the periods immediately before and after the anaesthetic from those of possible awareness. Some patients complain of dreams, which may or may not mean that they have had awareness. Other patients believe that they were unconscious for many hours postoperatively until after they reached their room on the ward and yet are able to describe events from the Recovery Room.

Patients who have suffered awareness may not be able to describe what happened yet they are very distressed. Reactions may include nightmares, inability to sleep and other sleep disturbances, anxiety, panic attacks, and depression. Some patients have reported that they thought that they were crazy, as did relatives, friends, and even the family doctor. Explaining what probably occurred is the first step in helping these patients to overcome the severe psychological distress and trauma that some have suffered from no one believing that they were awake during the procedure.

WILL I WAKE UP AFTER THE ANAESTHETIC?

You will 'wake up' afterwards unless there is a major complication with either the operation or the anaesthetic, or with some underlying condition. Some patients are given sedatives and painkillers that keep them sedated even after emergence from the anaesthetic. These drugs do not prevent you from waking up. Failure to regain consciousness is a sign of brain damage, and can be due to a direct effect of surgery on the brain, a lack of blood or oxygen to the brain, or a major chemical disturbance in the body, such as very low thyroid function. The risk of such a complication is generally considered to equal that of the risk of death during anaesthesia—that is, very low.

Your anaesthetist is continuously monitoring your blood pressure and the amount of oxygen in your blood. This is to ensure an adequate supply of oxygen to the brain and all other organs. Most often, brain damage is due to an interruption in the planned delivery of oxygen—for example, misplacement of the breathing tube in the oesophagus rather than in the windpipe, or unrecognised accidental disconnection of the ventilator. Current monitoring of carbon dioxide (by end-tidal capnography) and oxygen (by pulse oximetry) is intended to provide faster detection of problems and prevention of complications. Your anaesthetist is also prepared to deal with the consequences of surgical problems, such as sudden or large loss of blood.

COULD I HAVE A STROKE DURING THE ANAESTHETIC?

Even more rare than damage to all of the brain is the risk of a stroke or damage to part of the brain. A stroke occurs when there is decreased blood flow to a part of the brain, from blockage of a vessel by a clot, by an air bubble, or by haemorrhage. Certain patients are more at risk than others—for example, those undergoing cardiac surgery. Patients who have had a recent stroke or cerebrovascular accident (CVA) probably should not undergo elective operations (unrelated to their brain or to blood vessels of the neck) for several weeks. Unfortunately, if a patient suffers a stroke during an operation, the risk of death as a result of the stroke is high.

DO ANAESTHETIC DRUGS DAMAGE THE BRAIN?

Contrary to rumour, anaesthetic drugs are not toxic to the brain. If a patient is found to have brain damage postoperatively, then it is likely due to the operation (such as use of the heart-lung machine) or to some underlying condition (such as a blood clot). The role of the anaesthetic in causing brain damage is related to a lack of oxygen, usually from some problem with breathing, and not from a direct effect of the anaesthetic drugs.

AREN'T EPIDURALS DANGEROUS? CAN THEY CAUSE PARALYSIS?

This is a common question, especially from pregnant women. Unwanted effects of epidurals vary from mild to serious. Common side-effects include:

- **A feeling of weakness or heaviness in the legs:** This is the effect of the local anaesthetic and depends on which nerves (and how many) are blocked, as well as the strength of the local anaesthetic solution used.
- **A fall in blood pressure:** This is normally countered by the giving of some intravenous fluid, but occasionally requires drug treatment. The checking of your blood pressure is routine.
- **Difficulty passing urine:** This occasionally requires the temporary passage of a catheter into the bladder (with a small risk of introducing infection).
- **Backache:** This can occur after epidurals for labour, but it is also common in women who did not have an epidural.
- **Failure:** A small area of the pain is not blocked. Sometimes manipulation of the catheter can help, or the insertion of a second one. Occasionally the epidural has to be abandoned because of unsatisfactory pain relief.

- **Shivering or nausea:** This may be related to other drugs that are used, in addition to the local anaesthetics.

Complications include:

- **Puncture of the dura** (covering of the spinal cord and fluid) allowing a leak of spinal fluid into the epidural space: This may cause a severe headache, but it can be managed by bed rest, analgesics, and sometimes by having another epidural injection.
- **Nerve damage:** Sometimes temporary damage may occur to the spinal nerves, and it heals in about 12 weeks. The chance of this occurring is about 1 in every 3000 epidurals given for childbirth. It may be caused by nerve pressure during the labour itself and not by the epidural.
- **Injection of the local anaesthetic into a blood vessel:** This is very rare and can usually be avoided by the use of test doses of the drug.
- **Infection or blood clots:** These are also rare, providing care is taken to ensure that there is no skin infection and that the patient is not taking drugs to thin the blood.
- **Permanent paralysis:** This has been reported, but is exceptionally rare. The exact cause is usually not known.

Won't the epidural increase the chance that I'll need a Caesarean?

In the past, there was a suggestion that epidurals during childbirth decreased a woman's ability to push and prolonged the labour. This then led to a forceps delivery or Caesarean section. However, it is now well accepted that there is no significant effect from epidurals on the length of labour or on the chance of needing either a forceps delivery or a Caesarean section.

Modern approaches to the use of epidurals in labour include more active control by the mother over the birth process and the use of very low concentrations of drugs. As a result, many women are able to walk around in labour while still having some relief of pain. If labour is prolonged, for example because of a large baby, there may be a need for a forceps delivery or a Caesarean section. In such cases, the epidural inserted for pain relief during labour can then be used as the anaesthetic for the procedure.

Will the epidural affect my baby?

No, the drugs used for epidurals during childbirth do not have any effect on the baby. Babies born after the use of narcotic (morphine or pethidine) pain relief during labour are much more likely to show the effects of those drugs on their breathing.

HOW LIKELY AM I TO DIE?

There is a small risk of death while anaesthetised. It may be due to a complication of the operation, such as uncontrollable bleeding; to a worsening of some pre-existing disease, such as heart disease; or to a complication of the anaesthetic, usually from a problem with breathing leading to a lack of oxygen. Of these, the anaesthetic plays the smallest part in contributing to the risk of death. In fact, one study compared the risk of death due to surgery with that due to anaesthesia, in a large group of patients who were followed for the first thirty days after their operations. The risk of dying from the operation alone was 1 in 2860 while the risk of dying from the anaesthetic alone was 1 in 185,056. Currently, a fit, healthy, young to middle-aged patient undergoing straightforward elective surgery has a very small chance of dying due to a complication of the anaesthetic, probably less than 1 in 250,000.

When other factors, such as extremes of age, severe illness, and complicated or emergency surgery are added into the equation, the risk of death increases. However, we know from various studies that the overall risk of death from anaesthesia in most developed countries is still less than 1 in 60,000.

Although this number may seem very high to some, it is a remarkable improvement over the past century, when the risk of death from anaesthesia was about 1 in 100. Since then there has been a steady decrease in the number of deaths directly attributable to anaesthesia. For example, by 1948–52, the overall rate of death from (ether) anaesthesia was 1 in 820.

Not only has the death rate from anaesthesia (as a primary cause) fallen, but also the rate of death from anaesthesia as a contributing cause. The risk of death in which anaesthesia was a contributor has decreased to less than 1 in 15,000 anaesthetics.

Some of the anaesthetic factors that have contributed to a patient dying include incomplete preparation of the patient, inappropriate choice or use of an anaesthetic technique, and inadequate post-operative care.

This improvement in outcome is all the more remarkable considering the range of complex operations now performed and the very ill patients who undergo them. In fact, these operations are possible because of the advances in anaesthesia, such as the introduction of muscle relaxants.

One reason for this decrease in mortality is that the use of new monitoring equipment, such as pulse oximeters and capnography, leads to earlier recognition of problems during the anaesthetic, before the patient's condition has deteriorated. However, the death rate from anaesthesia was already decreasing before these monitors came into use. Other suggestions are that patients are better prepared for anaesthesia and surgery, and that training of both surgeons and anaesthetists has improved. The most likely explanation is that the decreasing death rate is due to a combination of all of these factors.

Of course, the risk of death from the anaesthetic alone must always be kept in perspective with that of the risk of the operation (for which the anaesthetic is given), the risk of dying after the operation, and the risk of various activities of daily life.

ARE CHILDREN MORE AT RISK?

Children having surgery fall into one of two groups. The biggest group is children who are otherwise well, apart from the condition for which they need a minor operation. A smaller group consists of children who are quite ill and about to undergo a major operation. In general, children do not suffer from many of the chronic illnesses that afflict adults, such as bronchitis, high blood pressure, heart disease, or the complications from consumption of alcohol and tobacco products. However, even children who are quite well may suffer from asthma (which is becoming increasingly common in Western society) and diabetes.

The risk of death in children undergoing anaesthesia is about the same as in a healthy adult. Children under one year of age, however, are at greater risk of complications, especially when cared for by anaesthetists who are not accustomed to managing children.

Most often, problems occur with breathing, either because the airway is not controlled or because breathing is not adequate. Compounding this is the fact that everything happens very quickly in children, including the development of complications.

WHAT IF A PROBLEM DOES OCCUR DURING THE ANAESTHETIC?

Anaesthetists are trained to manage complications. Thus, although complications occur rarely, your anaesthetist knows how to manage a reaction in the unlikely event that one does arise. Anaesthetists are starting to use realistic Operating Room simulators, in the same way that pilots use flight simulators to practise dealing with emergencies. In the forgiving environment of the simulator, artificial patients can be given the worst possible reactions—both anaesthetic and surgical—with which the anaesthetist and the rest of the Operating Room team must then cope. During these crises, of course, there is no risk to any real-life patients.

MY GRANDMOTHER'S SISTER DIED UNDER AN ANAESTHETIC. WHAT DOES THAT MEAN FOR ME?

Some conditions that run in families may cause problems during anaesthesia. Most can be easily and safely managed if the exact cause is known. If it was your grandmother's sister, there are several possibilities to consider. When did she have the anaesthetic? If it was many years ago, it might have been at a time when deaths under anaesthesia were more common and anaesthetists less knowledgeable.

If the anaesthetic was more recent, then one needs to know what type of operation she had. How fit was she? Was she ill and having an emergency operation? These are all factors that have some impact on the risks of undergoing anaesthesia and surgery.

If, however, her death was recent and unexpected and she was

a fit, healthy woman undergoing a routine procedure, your anaesthetist will want to know as much information as possible about
the events. With that information, and current knowledge about
inherited diseases, it may be possible to determine the cause of your
relative's death. In addition it may be necessary to order some
special tests to help in diagnosing the problem.

WHO WILL BE IN THE OPERATING ROOM?

The number of people present in the Operating Room depends on
the type of institution in which you have your operation or procedure. If your operation takes place in a small hospital or a private
clinic, you are looked after by your anaesthetist, your surgeon, and
two or three nurses, including one who helps the anaesthetist. If
your operation is in a large hospital, in which medical and nursing students are taught, other individuals could be present during
your operation, such as an anaesthetic trainee. If you are to undergo
a very complex operation, such as open-heart surgery, other doctors and technicians will be present, assisting the surgeon and
looking after various pieces of equipment, such as the heart-lung
machine.

Will I be exposed to the whole world?

Hospitals are notorious for dressing patients in skimpy gowns.
Most modern institutions are aware of the individual's rights to
personal modesty and it is often not necessary to be so stringent
about wearing hospital clothing. Children especially resent being
made to wear ill-fitting gowns. They should be allowed to wear
their own loose-fitting clothes.

Staff in the Operating Room are aware of the need for you to
be appropriately covered during surgery and anaesthesia. This is
not only for reasons of modesty but also to prevent loss of body
heat. You should try not to feel embarrassed by exposure to hospital and medical staff. To them, in the hospital setting, the human

body is an object of their professional expertise. However, at all times they endeavour to respect your desire for modesty. In particular, they observe any of your dress requirements related to your religious beliefs.

Chapter 10

Common complaints

'IT'S PROBABLY DUE TO THE ANAESTHETIC'

Many symptoms and complaints have been ascribed to anaesthesia over the years, often by well-meaning surgeons, nurses, family doctors, or helpful relatives. This most often occurs when the real cause of the problem is not obvious. In many cases the complaint is not actually related to the anaesthetic. However, if you have a concern, talk to your anaesthetist and seek an explanation.

ANXIETY

It is not uncommon for patients to feel stressed at the time of anaesthesia and surgery. Feeling stressed before going to the hospital is to be expected as it is not an event which we look forward to, nor do most of us experience it often enough to become more tolerant. Such stress can be managed and made less likely to result in aftereffects. You should discuss any concerns you might have with your surgeon, your anaesthetist and your family doctor. Above all, find out as much as you can about your illness and operation and take a role in your own management.

BACKACHE

Occasionally, a patient complains of localised pain in the back or in a joint. The usual cause is a decrease in muscle tone and manipulation of the joints while the patient was unconscious. Certain operations require patients to be placed in positions in which they would not normally find themselves. Patients at increased risk of

joint pain are those with arthritis and those undergoing long procedures. A quick check of the range of motion of your neck, arms,
and hips can go a long way to avoiding this sort of discomfort.
After the anaesthetic, rest, mild painkillers, and the application of
warmth ease this discomfort.

BRUISES

Patients often develop a small bruise at the site of insertion of the
intravenous cannula, in the back of the hand, in the forearm near
the wrist or, less often, in the bend of the elbow. These bruises can
become painful and may take a week or so to heal. Elderly patients,
and those with fragile skin and veins, bruise more easily and the
bruise often takes longer to disappear.

CHIPPED OR DAMAGED TEETH

Although anaesthetists are careful to avoid contact with the teeth,
damage may occur when metal or hard plastic instruments are used
to maintain an open airway, to help with insertion of the breathing (endotracheal) tube, or to suction out secretions from the mouth
and back of the throat. In most cases, damage occurs at the time
of tracheal intubation, in about one in every 1,000 intubations.
Dental damage may also occur when a patient bites down on an
oral airway during recovery from anaesthesia. The force generated
is enough to break both natural and restored teeth and has been
noted in between one-quarter and one-half of all reported cases of
dental damage.

Although human teeth are very strong, they become more brittle with age. Just as you may chip a tooth while eating, the same
may occur during intubation. Cosmetic dental work, with veneers,
crowns or bridges, is a particular concern, as these structures are
not as strong as natural teeth.

If you have had dental work, especially to your front teeth, then
you should inform your anaesthetist and discuss any concerns you
might have. You should also point out any teeth that are loose.
You may be able to lessen the risk of damage by having an alter-
native technique to general anaesthesia, such as regional anaesthesia

(if appropriate). However, in some cases, general anaesthesia with an endotracheal tube is necessary. Attempting to avoid tracheal intubation by using a mask may lead to other complications, such as aspiration of stomach contents into the lungs. Some anaesthetists try to prevent dental damage by removing the oral airway before their patients regain consciousness and replacing it with a soft short tube placed in one nostril. (This is known as a *nasal* airway.)

Should any of your teeth be damaged or lost during an anaesthetic or operation, or while you are in the Recovery Room, you will need emergency treatment. This includes reinsertion of the tooth (if appropriate) and emergency dental consultation (if available). Great effort should be made to locate any missing teeth, and you may need to have a chest X-ray to ensure that you have not inhaled a tooth. If you have and the tooth is not removed from your lung, there is a high risk of pneumonia.

Similarly, children may undergo anaesthesia while their first teeth are about to be lost. It is easy to dislodge them, and you should tell the anaesthetist which teeth are involved. Sometimes parents request the anaesthetist to remove a tooth that is about to fall out!

Adults with loose teeth should see a dentist, if possible, before their anaesthetic. The same suggestion applies if any of the teeth are badly broken or decayed. In addition, professional dental cleaning is recommended for patients who have gum disease, especially those who are booked to have a major operation.

COUGH

If you are a smoker or suffer from chronic bronchitis, it is not unusual for your cough to be a little worse after the anaesthetic. This is for two reasons. First, nicotine suppresses the normal mechanism by which the lungs expel mucus. During the course of the anaesthetic, some of the effect of the nicotine wears off, allowing the lungs to start to recover. Second, the breathing (endotracheal) tube and the anaesthetic gases may act as irritants in certain patients, provoking cough.

The best treatment for a smoker is to give up smoking at least six weeks before the anaesthetic. Patients with chronic bronchitis benefit from chest physiotherapy, and some may need adjustment of their bronchodilator medication, as well as a course of antibiotics. Both groups of patients may benefit from having active physiotherapy postoperatively.

EYE DAMAGE

Various types of eye damage may occur. The cornea or surface of the eye may be abraded when the eyelids are not completely closed, particularly if the face is covered with drapes or towels. Some anaesthetists choose to secure the eyelids closed with tape—although certain patients develop skin reactions and others complain of loss of eyelashes from removal of the tape. Other anaesthetists choose to insert a lubricating ointment into the eye—although eye infections have been reported if the ointment is contaminated. Some patients have complained of blurring of vision for a few hours postoperatively, because of the residual ointment. However, corneal damage may occur even if the eye is lubricated and taped shut. The presence of make-up, such as mascara, is potentially hazardous.

HALLUCINATIONS

These may be related to the use of a specific drug, called ketamine. This drug has particular attributes, which makes it extremely useful in patients with severe burns and other life-threatening injuries. It is widely known to cause a range of hallucinations that seem to be worse in adults. Sometimes the hallucinations can be prevented by using another drug such as Valium.

HAIR FALLING OUT OR NOT CURLING

Problems with the hair are often ascribed to the effects of the anaesthetic. However, there is no known relationship between these types of complications and any of the anaesthetic drugs. The effects are more likely due to stress and can occur as a result of stress without anaesthesia or surgery.

HOARSENESS

Patients may complain of a sore throat and hoarseness after anaesthetics for which insertion of a breathing tube (tracheal intubation) was required. These problems are generally short-lived.

Other patients complain of persistent hoarseness after an anaesthetic. When examined, they are occasionally found to have a vocal cord that does not work, secondary to damage of the nerve to the voice-box (larynx), the recurrent laryngeal nerve. This damage is often blamed on the anaesthetist from use of the laryngoscope and insertion of the breathing tube. However, this is rarely the cause of such damage, except when patients are ventilated (breathed for with a machine) for many days or weeks, as in the Intensive Care Unit. More commonly, damage to the nerve is the result of surgical manipulation or trauma, which may occur during thyroid or other neck operations. Other permanent voice changes are also more often due to surgical damage to another nerve, the external laryngeal nerve, than to the anaesthetic.

MUSCLE PAINS

Typically, patients complain the day after a general anaesthetic that they have pain in the muscles of the upper body, chest wall, back, and occasionally the lower body. These sensations are like the onset of influenza, although some patients complain about feeling as though they were 'run over by a truck'. Others complain that they have difficulty breathing or lifting the head from the pillow, or are unable to move. Commonly, these patients are young, have undergone minor procedures such as dental extractions, and went home on the day of the procedure, with resultant activity. Curiously, the problem does not affect children. The treatment is rest and mild analgesics. Symptoms should resolve after a few days.

The usual cause of this discomfort is termed 'sux myalgia' and results from the use of suxamethonium, a muscle relaxant. One might ask why this drug is used when it causes such pain (as well as other complications). Suxamethonium produces rapid onset of muscle relaxation, which is important when the anaesthetist needs to obtain rapid control of a patient's breathing. This may be the case in an emergency, when the patient has a full stomach and is at risk of regurgitating the stomach contents up the oesophagus and into the lungs.

NOSEBLEED

Sometimes, instead of passing the breathing (endotracheal) tube through your mouth, your anaesthetist chooses to pass it into one nostril and down the back of the throat and into your voice-box (larynx). This change in route may still involve insertion of the laryngoscope into your mouth, so that your anaesthetist can see where he or she is placing the tube. Some anaesthetists are able to pass the tube from the nostril into the larynx without looking— by listening to the change in breathing as the tube reaches the voice-box. Nasal intubation is normally used for operations around the face and mouth.

Insertion of the tube through the nostril often results in some bleeding from the nose after the tube is removed. This bleeding normally stops after a few minutes, although seeing the nose bleed may be distressing to family members.

SORE THROAT

A sore throat is quite common after having an anaesthetic or operation. Some of the soreness may be due to not being able to drink before the operation and then breathing dry anaesthetic gases. Many patients think that the breathing tube causes the sore throat. It is true that patients who have an endotracheal tube inserted are more likely to have a sore throat. Modern endotracheal tubes are much less irritating than the ones that were used in the past, and a lubricant is often used to make actual insertion of the tube easier. However, the soreness is probably more related to use of the laryngoscope, the instrument used by your anaesthetist to see where to place the tube. A sore throat is more likely in those patients in whom there were difficulties in seeing the larynx, such as those with prominent teeth, a small lower jaw, or a short neck. The soreness usually passes in a day or two and can be eased by a mild analgesic such as paracetamol (acetominophen), aspirin, or a soothing throat lozenge.

SORE TONGUE

The tongue may be bruised during the insertion of the endotracheal tube. This bruising is usually due to pressure from the laryngoscope. Occasionally the tongue may become sore and swollen after an oral airway has been used. In this case, the tongue may have been bunched up under the airway. As with a sore throat, a sore tongue usually only lasts for a day or two.

'GRAN IS NOT THE SAME ANY MORE'

Elderly patients, particularly those with progressive heart disease, high blood pressure, or a history of minor strokes, may suffer permanent changes after anaesthesia. This may be a result of a change in critical blood supply to certain parts of the brain, altering specific chemicals in the brain.

Blood supply to the brain may be subtly altered by a decrease in the amount of carbon dioxide in the blood and by slight changes in blood pressure. Many anaesthetic drugs have side-effects which can alter blood flow, although modern drugs are less likely to produce these effects. Even though all aspects of the circulation are carefully monitored during an anaesthetic, sometimes changes can occur.

Families may notice that the relative has undergone a minor personality change or a loss of recent memory. These changes are difficult to predict and largely impossible to prevent. In fact, some changes may be due to the fact that the patient has been taken from familiar surroundings to the disruptive environment of the hospital, where noise is common and sleep is disturbed. Usually patients recover completely, once they return to their home and their normal routines.

Chapter 11

Possible complications of anaesthesia

Although anaesthesia is safer than in the past, complications do occur. One large study showed that about 10 per cent of patients experienced some problem after the anaesthetic, which could be as major as inflammation of the liver (hepatitis) or as minor as muscle soreness. The most frequent complications are nausea, vomiting, and sore throat, which are described in chapter 10. Major non-fatal complications are most likely to be diagnosed by a doctor, nurse, or other health care worker. The following list describes some of these, as well as other problems. This list is selective and does not include all complications.

AMOROUS ADVANCES

On rare occasions patients awakening from anaesthesia make amorous advances towards or statements about their doctors or nurses. This may lead to embarrassment (should the patient recall what he or she said) or potential litigation or even criminal charges (should the patient actually believe that sexual impropriety occurred).

It should be noted, however, that the statements of alleged sexual impropriety after anaesthesia are not specific to any one drug. Similar allegations can be found in the earliest descriptions of anaesthetic practice, more than a hundred and fifty years ago. This type of behaviour is due to temporary loss of some inhibitions, not unlike that occasionally seen with alcohol intoxication. Recovery Room nurses are well aware of the potential for such reactions. They are trained to respond in a manner that does not cause embarrassment to anyone.

ANAESTHETIC DISEASES

Some patients develop complications because of the interaction of specific anaesthetic drugs with a pre-existing condition. There are very few 'anaesthetic diseases'—that is, specific diseases for which anaesthetic drugs must be carefully selected so as to minimise the risk of problems. However, these diseases do exist. The following brief description of two of these conditions is not meant to replace a more definitive source of information.

Malignant hyperthermia or malignant hyperpyrexia

First recognised in Australia in 1960, malignant hyperthermia or malignant hyperpyrexia (MH) consists of an unexplained rise in body temperature and muscle rigidity during anaesthesia, due to a massive increase in metabolism. Consumption of oxygen and production of carbon dioxide also rise markedly. Predisposition to malignant hyperthermia is an inherited condition and occurs in about 1 in 40,000 patients. It is triggered after exposure to specific anaesthetic drugs—the volatile anaesthetic agents (such as isoflurane) and suxamethonium. Triggering may occur on the first exposure to these drugs or even after repeated and uncomplicated anaesthetics.

Treatment of an episode of MH consists of stopping the triggering drug, stopping the operation if possible, and administering a drug called dantrolene. This is the only specific drug treatment for this syndrome; without it, about half of all patients who suffer a malignant hyperthermia reaction die. Other treatment is also important, in the form of extra oxygen, cooling, and resuscitative drugs and fluids.

Currently, the only test for MH is one performed on a piece of biopsied muscle, although unfortunately some tests appear to show that the patient has the condition when in fact the patient does not. (This is known as a 'false positive' test result.) The patient and close relatives should all be tested. A patient who has had an MH reaction or a positive test should obtain some form of Medic-Alert notification and carry this at all times.

If a patient with known MH requires an operation, the Operating Room should be specially prepared. No volatile anaesthetic agents should be used in the room for 12 hours and, if possible, then the patient should be scheduled as the first case of the day. A 'safe' technique should be used. This consists of avoiding the known triggering agents and is not difficult to achieve. Drugs that are considered safe include nitrous oxide, thiopentone, propofol, midazolam, narcotics, muscle relaxants such as curare or vecuroniun, and any of the local anaesthetic drugs. The patient's condition, including temperature, should be carefully monitored as with any general anaesthetic. This should continue into the postoperative period. Some patients have been reported to have a reaction after a 'safe' anaesthetic, but these reactions apparently have not been severe.

Plasma cholinesterase deficiency

Plasma cholinesterase deficiency or pseudocholinesterase deficiency (PChD) is an enzyme deficiency that affects the metabolism of some anaesthetic drugs, thus lengthening their action. These drugs include certain types of local anaesthetic agents and suxamethonium. It is important to remember that having PChD does not mean that the patient is 'allergic' to these drugs, but simply that the drug takes longer to wear off.

If a patient with PChD is given suxamethonium, the muscle relaxation from the drug may last for several hours, instead of a few minutes. During this time, the patient is unable to move or breathe spontaneously, and requires artificial ventilation. Sedation, to make the period of the profound weakness less unpleasant, is also important while the action of the drug wears off.

PChD may be inherited and is found in less than 0.01 per cent of the population. The condition may also occur in patients with liver failure and certain tumours, as well as in those exposed to specific drugs, such as ecothiopate, and to certain insecticides. Some women at the end of pregnancy may develop a very mild form of PChD, which disappears after the birth of the baby. The enzyme deficiency can be confirmed by a special blood test.

BLINDNESS

Blindness after both general and regional anaesthesia is rare, but it can occur. Loss of vision may result from pressure on the eye.

It may be that the arteries at the back of the eye (retina) become compressed, thus depriving the eye of oxygen. Smokers are more at risk than are nonsmokers, because nicotine constricts or narrows arteries, further depriving the eye and the brain of oxygen. Temporary blindness may also occur after spinal anaesthesia for resection of the prostate gland in men. This is due to the effect of a special chemical in the fluid placed in the bladder by the surgeon during the course of the operation. (See also 'Eye damage', p. 160.)

BLOOD CLOTS

Certain patients are at increased risk of having blood clots—for example, those taking oral contraceptives or hormone replacement. Certain surgical procedures also increase the risk of clots, such as operations that last several hours or are on the lower part of the body. In general, anaesthetics do not increase the risk of having a blood clot.

HALOTHANE HEPATITIS

This is a very rare liver complication, and is most often diagnosed in women who are obese and aged between fifty and sixty. Patients have often had a halothane anaesthetic in the month immediately before the halothane anaesthetic that triggers the condition. The patient usually starts to develop problems about a week later. Complaints include being unwell, having no appetite, being nauseated, having pain in the upper part of the abdomen, having a fever, being jaundiced, and occasionally having a rash and painful joints. In the most severe form, the patient rapidly develops liver failure, which may be fatal. The problem is thought to be an autoimmune reaction, and testing for antibodies to halothane is possible. Today, this drug is hardly ever used in adults but is still used in children because the risk of hepatitis is thought to be very low. Hepatitis has been reported exceedingly rarely after the use of other volatile anaesthetics.

HEART ATTACKS

It is possible to suffer a heart attack during the course of an anaesthetic. However, if one does occur, it is more likely to be on the second or third day after the operation. The risk of having a heart attack or myocardial infarction (MI) is very low, but patients who have previously suffered an MI should not have elective surgery during the first six months afterwards. Other patients at risk are those with severe hardening of the arteries of the neck (carotids).

NERVE DAMAGE

Almost any nerve can be damaged. Nerves of the face may be damaged by pressure from the anaesthetic breathing circuit or from the anaesthetist's fingers holding the face mask on and the chin forward. The most common nerve injury is to the ulnar nerve at the elbow, from compression against a hard surface. In general, the prevention of nerve damage is by careful positioning and padding of the patient during anaesthesia. In the past, the cause of postoperative nerve damage was always thought to be due to improper positioning of the patient; however, some patients who develop nerve damage have been found to have a pre-existing problem.

PNEUMOTHORAX

In this condition, air (or another gas) enters the normally empty space between the lungs and the chest wall. If not detected and treated, this can be life-threatening as the gas expands and compresses the heart and the major blood vessels in the chest, preventing blood from entering or leaving. Most often a patient has a small but undiagnosed leak in the lining of the lung. This leak increases with the use of artificial ventilation. The problem may occur spontaneously in those with congenital swellings (bullae) of the lungs or in asthmatics. In addition, the lining of the lung may be accidentally punctured by some injections around the neck or in the chest region.

WHEEZING

Patients with asthma or chronic obstructive lung disease (COLD) and smokers may develop wheezing or bronchospasm. Wheezing may also occur in previously healthy patients during an allergic reaction due to drugs or blood products or after aspiration of gastric contents. Wheezing may occur after such procedures as insertion of the breathing tube. When wheezing occurs, the flow of air is reduced, especially when breathing out (exhaling). Commonly, wheezing is easily treated by deepening the anaesthetic, removing the stimulus, or use of drugs such as salbutamol, aminophylline, or steroids. For particularly severe reactions, adrenaline may be required.

Chapter 12

If you think something has gone wrong

IS THERE A PROBLEM?

Do anaesthetics actually cause problems? Anaesthetics are not treatments in themselves. Patients do not go into hospital to have an anaesthetic, but to have an operation for which they need an anaesthetic. As a result, any complication is usually regarded as an unwanted effect. Many anaesthetists recognise that most problems in anaesthesia relate to a complex set of factors, including the patient's condition, human error, equipment, and the environment in which the operation is performed—the hospital and the regulatory agencies. Thus, perfect outcome after anaesthesia is unlikely to be achieved in every case.

Patients, too, have changed their thinking about anaesthetics. When any operation carried a high risk of death from shock, blood loss, and infection, patients who did survive counted themselves lucky. For example, Dr Samuel Johnson, the famous writer of the 1700s, celebrated the anniversary of his surviving an operation to remove a stone from his bladder. Today, with certain procedures described as 'virtually problem-free', patients are more likely to speak up about any complaint that they have.

One factor that makes it hard to determine if patients have suffered even minor complications is the difficulty with follow-up. Many patients are discharged home the same day. Patients who have had major operations may be sent to a smaller facility to recover. It is therefore more difficult for anaesthetists to see patients postoperatively. Anaesthetists are dependent on patients letting them know if there has been an unexpected problem, or upon the surgeon to relay such information. Unfortunately, such communication frequently does not take place. In some facilities, patients who remain in hospital are routinely visited or given questionnaires about their anaesthetic care. Other facilities telephone patients within a day or two of the anaesthetic and operation to determine how things have gone, or patients are given telephone numbers that can be used 24 hours a day in order to contact an anaesthetist.

Another factor to remember is that complications rarely result from the anaesthetic alone. As stated above, patients do not come into hospital to have an anaesthetic but to have an operation. In addition, the patient may have any number of medical problems before the operation. Large studies that have followed up patients after anaesthesia and surgery have shown that the two factors which are responsible for approximately 90 per cent of deaths are the patient's disease(s) and the surgical operation.

Although an anaesthetist may be able to influence a patient's condition through careful preoperative assessment and management, the same is not possible for the surgical factors. For example, the risk of complications increases with the duration of the surgical procedure. If an operation takes longer than about three to four hours, the patient has an increased chance of developing heart and lung problems. As a general rule, few patients die from the anaesthetic alone. Only about 10 per cent of patients suffer some other kind of anaesthetic-related complication, nearly all of them minor.

IF YOU THINK SOMETHING HAS GONE WRONG

Although the anaesthetic may not be the major contributor to how you feel after an operation, if you think something has gone wrong with your anaesthetic, it is very important to sort this out right away. Don't wait twenty years until you suddenly find that you need to have another operation.

Ask to speak to your anaesthetist or to another anaesthetist. Ask to have the anaesthetic record reviewed and, if possible, get the anaesthetist to show you the record and explain what each notation means.

If the anaesthetist suggests that you have special tests, have them done. These tests could include those for allergy; for plasma (or pseudo) cholinesterase; or for malignant hyperthermia (see chapter 11). Once the results are available, ask to have a copy that you may keep in your purse or wallet, or in the glove compartment of your car.

If your test results are positive, your anaesthetist may recommend that you obtain a Medic-Alert bracelet or similar type of medical information system. These are particularly useful if you become incapacitated and unable to explain your condition to the anaesthetist or to other doctors.

Above all, do not be afraid to find out what happened. Some patients worry for years that 'something dreadful happened to me during my anaesthetic', and put off having another needed operation. Visiting an anaesthetist and having the previous worrying events explained and demystified has freed these patients from unnecessary concerns.

Appendix 1
What you can do to help

FOR YOURSELF

- Get a little fitter. Even a regular walk will work wonders.
- Don't smoke—ideally, give it up six weeks before surgery.
- Drink less alcohol.
- Eat a healthy diet. Try to lose a little weight if you are overweight. Vitamin supplements may be appropriate.
- You may find relaxation exercises or tapes to be helpful.
- Continue to take any drugs that have been prescribed, but remember to tell your anaesthetist and surgeon.
- If you are taking aspirin, consult your surgeon or anaesthetist about whether or not you should stop taking it two weeks before surgery.
- If you are taking oral contraceptives, keep taking them, but tell your surgeon and anaesthetist.
- If you have any serious health problem, contact your anaesthetist or surgeon to see whether you need additional or different medicine or whether you need to see another specialist, such as a physician.
- If you have a cold or flu in the week before surgery, contact your anaesthetist or surgeon to find out if your anaesthetic and procedure or operation should be postponed.
- If you are anxious and have any questions, contact your anaesthetist to discuss them, or make an appointment to see him or her before admission.
- Learn about what is to be done. Talk to a friend or someone who has been through the procedure. Go to the library or check the Internet, for some of the references which we recommend in Further Information.

FOR YOUR CHILD

- Tell your child what is to happen. Above all, tell the truth.
- The length of preparation depends on age. Children under four years require preparation of a few hours. Those aged four to six need to be prepared for a day or two, while children over six may require several days to a week.
- Parental anxiety translates to the child, so parents need to have their questions answered by asking the anaesthetist and surgeon.
- Books, videos, preadmission clinics, and other activities, such as play-acting, may aid preparation.
- Open and truthful discussion is the key to successful preparation of the child for surgery and anaesthesia.

WHAT YOU SHOULD TELL YOUR ANAESTHETIST

- How healthy you are, and whether you have had any recent illnesses.
- Information about previous operations and anaesthetics.
- Any allergies and any abnormal reactions to drugs.
- Any history of asthma, bronchitis, heart problems, or other medical conditions.
- Whether or not you are taking any drugs at present— including tobacco or alcohol. If any are prescribed, bring them with you.
- If you are taking the contraceptive pill.
- If you have been taking aspirin.
- If you have any loose teeth, wear dentures, or have caps or plates.
- If you are concerned about anything in particular.

I don't want to bother the doctor

Whatever the cause, your anaesthetist needs to know any information that might influence the safety of your anaesthetic. You must let him or her know, even if it seems unimportant or embarrassing.

IF YOU ARE ADMITTED ON THE DAY OF SURGERY

- Follow fasting instructions. They are for your safety while undergoing anaesthesia.
- Do not drink any alcohol for the 24 hours before surgery.
- Do not smoke on the morning of surgery.
- If you normally take medications in the morning, do so with a small sip of water, unless instructed otherwise.
- Take your regular medications with you to hospital.
- Remove nail polish because this may interfere with the pulse oximeter (the monitor that senses how much oxygen is in your blood).
- Remove contact lenses, hairpieces, and false eyelashes.

IF YOU ARE DISCHARGED ON THE SAME DAY AS YOUR OPERATION

- Arrange with someone to escort you home from hospital.
- Arrange for someone to stay with you overnight.
- Do not, for a period of 24 hours:
    - drive a car or ride a motorcycle, bicycle or horse
    - use power appliances or tools
    - cook or pour hot liquids
    - drink alcohol
    - sign legal or financial documents.

Appendix 2
Questions to ask

These are questions for you to ask your anaesthetist before your operation, although you may not want to use them all.

CHOICE OF ANAESTHETIC

- Do I have a choice about the type of anaesthetic I will have?
- Do I have to have a general anaesthetic, or can I have the procedure done under a local anaesthetic or a regional anaesthetic?
- What are the complications and risks with each type of anaesthetic that I can have for this procedure?
  - local
  - regional
  - general
- What can I do to prevent or minimise these?
- Does my condition make me more likely to suffer any complications from the anaesthetic?
  - local
  - regional
  - general

BEFORE MY ANAESTHETIC

- Do I have to have any tests?
- Do I need a sedative:
  - the night before the operation?
  - the day of the operation?
- What should I do about my medication?
  - Are there any I should not take?
  - When should I take them?

- When should I stop:
  - eating solid food?
  - drinking clear liquids?
- Can I leave:
  - my dentures/bridgework in?
  - my hearing aid in?
  - my glasses on?
  - my underwear on?
- Can my family come with me to the Operating Room?

IN THE OPERATING ROOM

- What will I see, hear and feel in the Operating Room?
- Who will be looking after me?
- If I have a regional anaesthetic, then can I, or do I have to, have any sedative drugs during the operation?
- How long will I be there?

IN THE RECOVERY ROOM

- What will I see, hear and feel in the Recovery Room?
- Will I be sick?
  - How can this be treated?
- Will I be in pain?
  - How can this be treated?
- How long will I be there?
- Can my family see me?

ON THE WARD

- How will I feel when I get back to the ward?
- Will I be sick?
  - How can this be treated?
- Will I be in pain?
  - How can this be treated?

- When can I have something:
  - to eat?
  - to drink?

AT HOME

- When can I go home?
- Will I need to take any tablets or other medications after the anaesthetic?
  - If yes, will these medications have any side-effects?
  - What can I do to prevent or minimise these?
- Will I have any limitations to what I can do after my anaesthetic?
- When can I go back to work or to school?

Appendix 3
A brief history of anaesthesia

The modern anaesthetic era is only just over a hundred and fifty years old. Successful anaesthesia for surgery was first demonstrated in 1846. Before that, the few operations that were possible were carried out either with no pain relief or after a dose of opium and/or alcohol.

There were many attempts to relieve pain throughout the centuries. Early examples include loss of consciousness produced by blows to the patient's head or by compression of the carotid arteries (in the neck). In the Middle Ages, elaborate potions included alcohol and various plant extracts such as mandrake root. Opium was widely used, particularly in China, and the first *intravenous* injection of opium was made in the 1660s. Pain relief in an arm or a leg was produced by squeezing the nerves in the upper part of the limb and also by applying cold water, ice, or snow. Hypnotism became popular as a means of pain relief and medical treatment during the late eighteenth and early nineteenth centuries.

The seventeenth and eighteenth centuries were marked by a rapid increase in knowledge of how the heart and lungs worked, as well as the properties of many gases. In 1799, Sir Humphrey Davy suggested the use of nitrous oxide to produce pain relief. Twenty-five years later, Dr Henry Hickman described the use of carbon dioxide to produce loss of consciousness, while Horace Wells first used nitrous oxide for extraction of teeth in 1844.

Although Paracelsus described the effects of *ether* on animals in 1540, the first use of this drug for general anaesthesia in humans was in 1842 by Drs Long and Clark. On 16 October 1846, Dr William Morton gave the first public demonstration of ether anaesthesia in Boston. The operating room where this occurred, known

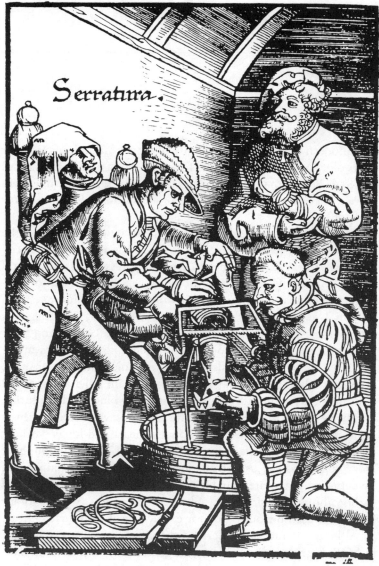

Figure 10   A surgical operation before anaesthesia.

as the Ether Dome, is preserved intact at the Massachusetts General Hospital. This major advance in the relief of human suffering spread rapidly, and the first use in the United Kingdom, Canada, Australia, and New Zealand followed soon thereafter.

'ANAESTHESIA'

A few weeks after the famous ether demonstration, Oliver Wendell Holmes popularised the word 'anaesthesia'. He used the word to describe 'insensibility—more particularly to objects of touch', as produced by ether. The word had been used previously to describe simply any lack of feeling—for example, that due to a nerve problem. Holmes also introduced such combinations of words as 'anaesthetic state' and 'anaesthetic agent'.

Professor James Young Simpson of Edinburgh introduced *chloroform* in 1847. He also described the first anaesthetic death in 1848, the patient being a young girl named Hannah Greener. She was the first of many who suffered sudden heart failure under chloroform. In London, John Snow led the way in analysing complications after anaesthesia and surgery, with a careful evaluation of postoperative deaths. He attempted to modify his practice by referring to what he had learned from previous cases.

Anaesthesia produced by *nerve block*, or *regional anaesthesia*, became possible after cocaine was isolated from the coca plant in 1860. Dr Karl Koller first produced anaesthesia of the skin and mucous membranes in 1884. In New York in 1885, Dr Corning gave the first spinal anaesthetic and then the first *epidural* anaesthetic in 1901.

General anaesthesia became more pleasant for patients when *Pentothal* or sodium thiopentone came into use in the late 1930s. Muscle relaxation using curare was first demonstrated in humans in 1942, allowing a lighter depth of general anaesthesia than had been previously possible. In the 1950s, the investigation of halogenated hydrocarbons as nonflammable, highly potent anaesthetic agents resulted in the introduction of halothane and the disappearance of ether and chloroform from most operating rooms.

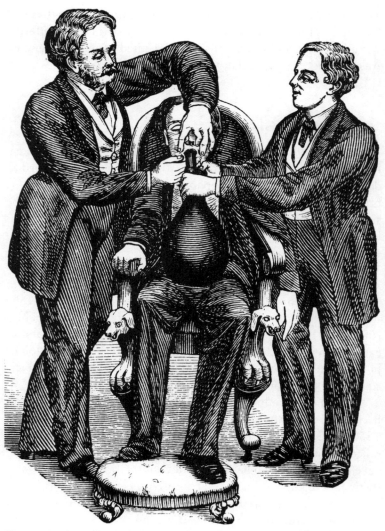

Figure 11   Anaesthesia in the 1850s. The patient is being given nitrous oxide to breathe from a bladder or leather bag.

THE MODERN ERA

The modern era of anaesthesia began in the 1960s, with the development of new drugs and the availability of new monitoring techniques and equipment. As more information became available to the anaesthetist as to what was happening to the patient and in the anaesthetic delivery system, so anaesthetists began to look more closely at safety and refinement of techniques. Surgery was extended to increasingly complex procedures on patients who might previously have been denied operations on the basis of age or illness. Anaesthesia also led the way in analysis of 'critical incidents' or the study of near-misses, a process only now being extended to other areas of medical care.

The end of the twentieth century saw major advances in everyday anaesthesia, including the contributions of computer technology, microelectronics, and advances in drugs. Anaesthesia is now tailored to each individual patient, and whether you are ten weeks premature or a hundred years old, whether you are sick or well, there has never been a safer time to undergo anaesthesia.

Glossary

Acute pain. Pain of sudden onset, especially after surgery or injury, or associated with illness.

Adrenaline. A naturally occurring chemical produced in the body in response to stress. When given as a drug it causes increases in heart rate and blood pressure. Adrenaline is also used as a treatment for severe allergic reactions.

Airway. The part of the body through which the air passes on its way to the lungs. The 'upper airway' usually refers to the mouth and throat as far down as the voice-box (larynx); the 'lower airway' refers to the air passages below the larynx. 'Airway' also refers to a tube placed through the mouth or nose to facilitate the free movement of air, oxygen, or anaesthetic gases.

Anaesthesia (anesthesia). The state of loss of sensation.

Anaesthetic. Drug or agent used to induce or maintain anaesthesia. Also used to refer to the state of anaesthesia.

Anaesthetic machine. The equipment used to deliver the anaesthetic gases and to support the monitors and breathing systems used during anaesthesia.

Anaesthetic record. The written or computer-generated record of the process and events of a particular anaesthetic. Details noted include drugs and doses; measurements such as heart rate and blood pressure; amount (or percentage) of oxygen delivered; fluids given and blood lost; and surgical events.

Anaesthetic technician. A trained health worker who assists the anaesthetist.

Anaesthetist (anesthesiologist, anaesthesiologist). The person, usually a doctor, who administers the anaesthetic.

Analgesic. Drug used to relieve pain.

Anaphylactic, anaphylactoid. Severe allergic reaction requiring immediate treatment. May be fatal.

Antagonist. A drug that acts within the body to counteract the effect of another drug.

Anti-emetic. A drug that is used to prevent or treat nausea and vomiting.

Arthroscope. A small fibre-optic probe used to look at the inside of joints.

Aspiration. The inhalation of stomach contents into the lungs.

Awareness. The state of being aware of events during general anaesthesia and surgery.

Biopsy. A piece of tissue removed from a part of the body for various tests and examination under a microscope.

Breathing system. A series of hoses and chambers that contain and deliver the gas and vapour mixtures that are breathed by the patient during anaesthesia.

Bronchoscopy. The process of looking into parts of the upper airway (larynx) and the lung (trachea and air passages (bronchi)) by means of a fibre-optic probe.

Bronchus (plural: bronchi). The major air passage of the lungs.

Caesarean section. The operation to deliver a baby through the abdomen rather than allow it to be born via the birth canal.

Cannula (plural: cannulae). Sometimes called a catheter. A short hollow plastic tube that can be placed into a blood vessel for sampling blood or giving fluid or drugs directly into the bloodstream.

Cardiologist. A doctor who specialises in diseases of the heart.

Cataract. A change in the lens of the eye where the lens becomes opaque.

Caudal. A type of epidural anaesthetic, but restricted to the lower end of the spinal cord.

Chart. See 'hospital record'.

Chloroform. One of the earliest anaesthetic agents, used as a vapour and having a sweet smell. It has a high risk of severe side-effects and death.

Chronic pain. Pain that persists for a long time, usually more than two or three months.

Circuit. See 'breathing system'.

Colostomy. The result of an operation, usually for bowel cancer, in which the lower end of the bowel is relocated to an artificial opening on the front of the abdomen.

Faeces are collected into a special plastic bag and emptied as necessary.

Cricoid pressure. External pressure applied to the cricoid cartilage of the windpipe or trachea in order to compress the oesophagus and minimise the chance of regurgitation.

CT scan. A specialised X-ray which produces multiple images taken in a 360-degree circle. The patient is required to lie still in the centre of the scanner for several minutes.

Deep vein thrombosis (DVT). Clotting and inflammation of the veins, usually in the calves of the legs. There is a risk that some of the clot may dislodge and travel in the bloodstream back to the heart and lungs, where it may cause major blockage of the blood flow. DVT is more common in the elderly, females, smokers, obese patients, and those having major surgery for cancer. Prevention is mainly by the use of anti-clotting agents and having the patient get out of bed and start walking as soon as possible after the operation.

Disorientation. A state of confusion or inability to know where one is, what the time is, and even who one is.

Droperidol. A drug used to reduce the chance of nausea and vomiting. Droperidol may also cause some unpleasant psychological reactions.

Dysphoria. An unpleasant psychological reaction.

Elective. Not urgent (when referring to surgery).

Electrocardiograph (ECG or EKG). A monitor that measures the small electrical impulses from the heart and displays them on a screen.

Emergence. The phase of anaesthesia during which patients 'emerge' from the anaesthetised state to regain at least some control over their functions. After emergence, patients are transferred to a special area where continued recovery occurs under the care of a nurse, as delegated by the anaesthetist.

Emergency. Requiring urgent attention to avoid the risk of damage or death to the patient or body part.

Endobronchial intubation. Passage of an endotracheal tube further than usual down the trachea and into one of the two bronchi (major air passages of the lungs).

Endoscopy. The process of using a fibre-optic scope to observe and operate in parts of the body not otherwise accessible without invasive surgery.

Endotracheal intubation. The placement of a breathing tube into the trachea or windpipe.

Ephedrine. See 'adrenaline'.

Epidural. Epidural anaesthesia refers to the placement of drugs into the epidural space. This is the space that surrounds the spinal cord and its covering layers, through which the spinal nerves pass as they connect to other nerves leading to and from all parts of the body.

Epiglottis. The flap or 'trapdoor' over the opening to the voice-box (larynx).

Ether. An anaesthetic drug administered as a vapour. It was one of the first anaesthetic agents used and has a very pungent smell. It has now been replaced by safer and more acceptable drugs.

Euphoria. Pleasant psychological reaction. A 'high'.

Extubation. The removal of the endotracheal tube from the trachea.

Fibroids. Benign swellings in the muscular wall of the uterus.

Full stomach. A term used to describe the potential for the stomach to have failed to empty properly before the anaesthetic is started. This is most common in cases where the bowel is obstructed, or the patient has been involved in an accident (even a minor one) between the time of last eating and the time of surgery.

General anaesthesia. Anaesthesia applied to the whole body. A state of controlled unconsciousness.

Goitre. A swelling of the thyroid gland, which is situated in the front of the neck.

Haemoglobin. The chemical contained in red blood cells that is responsible for carrying oxygen.

Haemorrhoidectomy. The operation to remove haemorrhoids (dilated veins in the rectum or anus).

Hernia. An outpouching of the lining of the abdominal cavity, through a weakness in the overlying muscular layers.

Hiatus hernia. A widening of the normal space between the abdomen and the chest through which the oesophagus passes. As a result, part of the stomach slides into the chest, and acid from the stomach is able to flow up the oesophagus, causing 'heartburn' (indigestion).

High Dependency Unit (HDU). See 'Intensive Care Unit'.

Hospital record. The files or records of a patient's admissions and treatments provided by a particular hospital.

Hypoxia. Insufficient oxygen in the bloodstream, sometimes caused by the breathing of a gas mixture with inadequate oxygen.

Hysterectomy. The operation to remove the uterus.

Incision. A cut into the surface of the body or an organ.

Induction. The process of starting the anaesthetic.

Induction agents. Drugs used to induce anaesthesia.

Informed consent. Consent for a procedure that is given by the patient or a responsible person, having understood the explanations and implications provided by the treating doctor.

Inhalation. The act of inhaling; that is, taking air or gas into the lungs by breathing.

Inhalational agents. Anaesthetic drugs administered as a vapour or gas and breathed in by the patient.

Intensive Care Unit (ICU). A specialised ward for the care of critically ill patients.

Internist. See 'physician'.

Intramuscular. Literally 'inside or within the muscle', referring to the site of injections.

Intraoperative. During the operation.

Intravenous (IV). Into the vein, by injection. Sometimes the word 'intravenous' refers to a cannula inserted into a vein as a means of injecting drugs intravenously. The cannula may or may not have a fluid infusion or intravenous line attached.

Intubation. The placement of a tube into a hollow space. In most cases this refers to the placement of an endotracheal tube into the larynx.

Laparoscope. A type of fibre-optic probe used when looking into or operating in the abdominal cavity.

Laryngeal mask airway (LMA). A device used to connect the breathing circuit to the patient's trachea without passing a tube through the larynx (voice-box). The LMA consists of a tube with an inflatable pad that encloses the larynx.

Laryngoscope. A device used to insert an endotracheal tube into the trachea. The laryngoscope consists of a long metal 'blade' with a light, which is inserted into the mouth of the anaesthetised patient so the anaesthetist can see the larynx.

Larynx. The site of the vocal cords. Commonly known as the voice-box or Adam's apple, it may be felt in the neck as a hard lump. The larynx connects the throat to the trachea.

Local anaesthesia. Anaesthesia applied to a part of the body, usually by blocking the transmission of nerve impulses in one or more nerves.

Local anaesthetics. Drugs, such as lidocaine, that are used to produce local or regional anaesthesia.

Lymph nodes. Part of the body's defence system, consisting of small glands that respond to infection by swelling up. They are often the sites to which cancer spreads.

Maintenance. The phase of anaesthesia between 'induction' and 'emergence'. This is the period during which the surgical or other procedure may be performed.

Malignant hyperthermia/hyperpyrexia (MH). A rare condition in which, after administration of certain triggering drugs, the patient develops an uncontrollable rise in temperature. The susceptibility is hereditary and the condition is treatable.

Mandible. The lower jaw.

Material risks. Risks that may occur and that represent serious complications.

Mediastinoscopy. The process of looking into the front part of the chest cavity, using a fibre-optic probe inserted at the bottom of the neck.

Meperidine. See 'pethidine'.

Monitored anaesthesia care. Care for a patient by an anaesthetist where a general anaesthetic is not administered.

Monitors. Devices that measure changes in some aspect of the patient's condition, such as heart rate, or of a piece of equipment—for example, concentration of oxygen delivered from the anaesthetic machine. (A car speedometer is a monitor of road speed.)

Morphine. A powerful painkilling drug.

Muscle relaxants. Drugs used to induce relaxation or weakening of muscles.

Myocardial infarction (MI). A heart attack. Specifically refers to the damage (infarction) caused by lack of blood supply to a section of the heart muscle (myocardium).

Narcotics. Painkilling drugs derived from opium, or related synthetic compounds.

Nasal. Pertaining to the nose.

Nasogastric tube. A narrow plastic tube inserted through one nostril, down the oesophagus and into the stomach.

Nerve block. The use of local anaesthetic around a nerve to block the passage of impulses down the nerve fibre.

Non-steroidal anti-inflammatory drugs (NSAIDs). These drugs provide pain relief and reduce inflammation, but are not members of the narcotic group of painkilling drugs.

NPO. 'Nil per os', i.e. 'nothing by mouth'—in other words, no food or drink.

Obstetricians. Doctors who specialise in the care of women during pregnancy and delivery.

Obstructive sleep apnoea (OSA). A condition where partial blockage to breathing in the mouth and at the back of the throat leads to short periods of interruption of breathing while asleep. Such breathing while asleep is usually noisy, as in snoring.

Oral. Pertaining to the mouth.

Palate. The roof of the mouth.

Patient-controlled analgesia (PCA). Pain relief with intravenous administration of narcotic analgesics, where the rate of administration is under the patient's control. A delivery system is programmed so that overdoses cannot be given.

Pentothal. A commonly used brand of thiopentone.

Peripheral. In an extremity, such as an arm or a leg. Opposite to 'central'.

Pethidine. A strong narcotic painkiller, such as morphine.

Phlebitis. Inflammation of the veins, usually confined to a small area.

Physicians. Doctors who specialise in internal medicine—that is, in diseases of the body not usually associated with the need for surgery. Also known as 'internists'.

Placenta. The organ that grows in the uterus with the developing baby and provides a connection with the mother, so that oxygen, carbon dioxide, and other nutrients and waste products can be exchanged between the mother's and baby's bloodstreams.

Polyps. Swollen lumps of tissue, usually in the nose or bowel.

Postoperative. After the operation.

Premedication. The administration of medication to a patient before anaesthesia. This medication may include drugs to relieve pain, sedatives, anti-emetics, or specific treatments, as well as the patient's normal medication(s).

Preoperative. Before the operation.

Propofol. A drug used for induction of anaesthesia. It is a white milky liquid and has been used since the late 1980s.

Pulse oximeter. A monitor that measures the saturation or percentage of oxygen in the bloodstream and the heart rate. The sensor probe is a simple wrap-around or peg-like device that is attached to a finger, toe, or earlobe.

Radiologist. A doctor who specialises in diagnosing illnesses and other conditions through the use of X-rays and other imaging techniques.

Rapid sequence induction. Rapid induction of anaesthesia because of a risk of vomiting or regurgitation.

Recovery Room. The area near the Operating Room to which a patient is transferred to continue recovery from both the anaesthesia and the surgery.

Regional anaesthesia. See 'local anaesthesia'.

Regurgitation. The passage of fluid or partially digested food back up the oesophagus from the stomach to the mouth. Regurgitation does not imply active vomiting.

Respiratory therapist. A trained health worker who specialises in the care of breathing, especially in severe illness.

Rheumatoid arthritis. An inflammatory condition of joints and tendons. Can be very painful and debilitating.

Sedation. A state of calmness, or the process of producing such a state. Usually achieved by the use of sedative drugs.

Sputum. Spittle or mucus and other material coughed up from the lungs.

Stress test. A test that may be performed to estimate the capacity of the heart and lungs to withstand additional stresses, such as those imposed by surgery.

Thiopentone. A drug used to induce anaesthesia.

Thyroid cartilage. The main cartilage of the larynx (voice-box). This is the hard lump known as the Adam's apple in the front of the neck.

Titrating. Adjusting the dose of a drug as it is being administered, according to the effect it has on the patient.

Toxicity. Liability to cause damage.

Trachea. The tube that connects the larynx to the lungs. Commonly known as the windpipe.

Tracheal intubation. See 'endotracheal intubation'.

Ultrasound. The use of sound waves to examine parts of the body. Commonly used during pregnancy to examine the state of the growing baby and the placenta.

Vena cava. The large vein draining venous (deoxygenated) blood from the lower half of the body back to the heart.

Ventilator. A mechanical device that acts on the breathing system to move gas into and out of the patient's lungs.

Further information

Many of these web sites provide links to other sites that may be of interest.

General
http://www.asahq.org/homepageie.html
http://www.cas.ca/anaesthesia/
http://www.anesthesia.org/public/public.html
http://www.asa.org.au/public/anaesnu.htm

Local and regional anaesthesia
http://www.oyston.com/anaes/local.html

Pain relief in labour and childbirth
http://www.anesthesia.org/public/guides/lpain01.html
http://www.soap.org/about.htm

Paediatric anaesthesia
http://www.crha-health.ab.ca/clin/anaesth/paed/paed.htm

Malignant hyperthermia/hyperpyrexia
http://www.mhassn.com/index.html

Methods of minimising blood transfusion
http://www.watchtower.org/library/g/2000/1/8/article_03a.htm

Index